Frontiers in Clinical Drug Research- HIV

(Volume 4)

Edited by

Atta-ur-Rahman, *FRS*

Honorary Life Fellow, Kings College, University of Cambridge, Cambridge, UK

General:

1. Any dispute or claim arising out of or in connection with this License Agreement or the Work (including non-contractual disputes or claims) will be governed by and construed in accordance with the laws of the U.A.E. as applied in the Emirate of Dubai. Each party agrees that the courts of the Emirate of Dubai shall have exclusive jurisdiction to settle any dispute or claim arising out of or in connection with this License Agreement or the Work (including non-contractual disputes or claims).
2. Your rights under this License Agreement will automatically terminate without notice and without the need for a court order if at any point you breach any terms of this License Agreement. In no event will any delay or failure by Bentham Science Publishers in enforcing your compliance with this License Agreement constitute a waiver of any of its rights.
3. You acknowledge that you have read this License Agreement, and agree to be bound by its terms and conditions. To the extent that any other terms and conditions presented on any website of Bentham Science Publishers conflict with, or are inconsistent with, the terms and conditions set out in this License Agreement, you acknowledge that the terms and conditions set out in this License Agreement shall prevail.

Bentham Science Publishers Ltd.
Executive Suite Y - 2
PO Box 7917, Saif Zone
Sharjah, U.A.E.
Email: subscriptions@benthamscience.net

BENTHAM SCIENCE

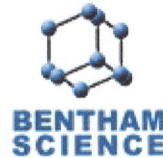

CONTENTS

PREFACE

The book series ***Frontiers in Clinical Drug Research-HIV*** presents important recent developments in the form of cutting edge reviews written by eminent authorities in the field. The chapters in this 4th volume are mainly focused on different types of HIV-1 inhibitors (integrase inhibitors, protease inhibitors, entry inhibitors, *etc.*), magnetic nanotherapeutics, and sexually transmitted co-infections.

Alluri and Ganguly in Chapter 1 discuss the design and synthesis of HIV-1 protease inhibitors based on a cyclic sulfonamide core structure. Sagar *et al.*, in chapter 2 discuss the importance of magnetic nanocarriers for delivering therapeutics which can exert changes at genetic levels. Chapter 3 by Watts *et al.*, describes the synthesis of currently FDA approved integrase inhibitor drugs and other HIV drugs developed through flow technology.

Chapter 4 by Yi-Qun Kuang focuses on the development and clinical progress on chemokine receptor-based HIV entry inhibitors. Cobucci *et al.*, in chapter 5, discuss the most prevalent co-infections found in HIV carriers and their epidemiology, clinical features and evidence-based treatments.

I am grateful to all the eminent scientists for their excellent contributions. I also express my gratitude to the editorial staff, particularly Mr. Mahmood Alam (Director Publication), Mr. Shehzad Naqvi (Editorial Manager Publications) and Ms. Fariya Zulfiqar (Manager Publications) for their hard work and persistent efforts.

Prof. Atta-ur-Rahman, *FRS*
Kings College
University of Cambridge
Cambridge
UK

List of Contributors

Ana Paula Ferreira Costa	Avenida Salgado Filho, Natal, RN, Brazil
Arti Vashist	Center for Personalized Nanomedicine/Institute of Neuroimmune Pharmacology, Department of Immunology, Herbert Wertheim College of Medicine, Florida International University, Miami, FL - 33199, USA
Ashit K. Ganguly	Stevens Institute of Technology, 1 Castle Point Terrace, Hoboken, NJ, USA
Faith Akwi	Nelson Mandela University, University Way, Port Elizabeth, 6031, South Africa
Madhavan Nair	Center for Personalized Nanomedicine/Institute of Neuroimmune Pharmacology, Department of Immunology, Herbert Wertheim College of Medicine, Florida International University, Miami, FL - 33199, USA
Marcos Gonzaga dos Santos	Avenida Salgado Filho, Natal, RN, Brazil
Omobolanle Janet Jesumoroti	Nelson Mandela University, University Way, Port Elizabeth, 6031, South Africa
Paul Watts	Nelson Mandela University, University Way, Port Elizabeth, 6031, South Africa
Ricardo Ney Oliveira Cobucci	Avenida Salgado Filho, Natal, RN, Brazil
Sesha S. Alluri	Stevens Institute of Technology, 1 Castle Point Terrace, Hoboken, NJ, USA
Vidya Sagar	Center for Personalized Nanomedicine/Institute of Neuroimmune Pharmacology, Department of Immunology, Herbert Wertheim College of Medicine, Florida International University, Miami, FL - 33199, USA
Yi-Qun Kuang	Center for Translational Medicine, Huaihe Clinical College, Huaihe Hospital of Henan University, Kaifeng, Henan, China

CHAPTER 1

Design and Synthesis of HIV-1 Protease Inhibitors

Sesha S. Alluri and **Ashit K. Ganguly**[*]

Stevens Institute of Technology, 1 Castle Point Terrace, Hoboken, NJ-07030, USA

Abstract: Human immunodeficiency virus (HIV-1) protease inhibitors play an important role as a part of the HAART (Highly Active Antiretroviral Therapy) treatment regimen for AIDS infection. The main cellular target for HIV-1 is helper T-lymphocytes that is critical to the immune system and renders individuals susceptible to opportunistic infections and tumors. According to World Health Organization, globally 36.9 million people are living with HIV-1 at the end of 2017 making HIV-1 a prime target for drug discovery.

HIV-1 belongs to the family 'retroviridae' that characteristically carry their genetic information in the form of ribonucleic acid (RNA). There are several drug targets that interfere with the life cycle of HIV-1 virus. Drugs such as enfuvirtide inhibit the entry of HIV-1 into the cell by interacting with CD4 receptors and co-receptors CCR5/CXCR4. Three key enzymes involved in the survival and replication of virus inside the host cell are reverse transcriptase, integrase, and protease. Once inside the host, the viral enzyme reverse transcriptase converts the viral RNA into proviral DNA. Azido thymidine (AZT) was the first reverse transcriptase inhibitor discovered. In the next step of viral replication, the proviral DNA is inserted into the host cell genome by the viral enzyme, HIV-1 integrase. Integrase inhibitors (*e.g.* raltegravir) block this step. Following integration, viral transcription factors cause the normal cellular machinery to produce multiple copies of viral m-RNA, which is transported from the nucleus back into the cytoplasm. In the cytoplasm, viral core proteins are produced as long chain polypeptides that are cleaved by the viral HIV-1 protease enzyme, into smaller polypeptides in order to become functional. HIV-1 protease inhibitors block this step and are considered as major breakthrough in AIDS research. Although there are several drug classes that inhibit the life cycle of HIV-1 virus at various stages, the major emphasis of this chapter will be on the discovery of linear sulfonamides such as darunavir which in particular is being very successfully used in the clinic. We shall also summarize the discovery from our laboratory of a novel class of cyclic sulfonamides as potent HIV-1 protease inhibitors.

The HIV-1 protease inhibitors represent one of the classic examples of structure-based drug design. The X-ray crystal structure of HIV-1 protease was determined in 1989 and several inhibitors were soon developed based on the configuration of the active site. Protease inhibitors such as saquinavir, ritonavir, indinavir, amprenavir, tipranavir, darunavir *etc.*, are successfully used for the treatment of AIDS patients. Today, new

[*] **Corresponding author Ashit K. Ganguly:** Stevens Institute of technology, 1 Castle Point Terrace, Hoboken, NJ-07030, USA; Tel: 201-216-3524; Email: akganguly1@aol.com

protease inhibitors are continuously being developed and designed because HIV-1 virus mutates quickly, and current medications are becoming increasingly ineffective.

In our published work, we have successfully discovered a novel class of HIV-1 protease inhibitors based on a cyclic sulfonamide core structure. HIV-1 protease inhibitors in clinical use such as amprenavir, tipranavir and darunavir possess sulfonamide moiety in their core structure. Unlike open chain sulfonamides used in the clinic, our compounds possess a conformationally restricted sulfonamide pharmacophore. Molecular modeling was used for the design of these inhibitors and the crucial step in their synthesis involved an unusual endo radical cyclization process.

Several analogs were synthesized in order to determine their structure activity relationship. X-ray crystallographic analysis confirmed the binding modes of our inhibitors to the HIV-1 protease enzyme. The structures of the novel inhibitors were further optimized to the picomolar affinities in the HIV-1 protease assay. More work remains to be done to determine whether these cyclic sulfonamides could be clinically useful.

Keywords: AIDS, Carbamates, Classes of HIV-1 Drugs, Cyclic Sulfonamides, HIV-1 Protease Inhibitors, Hydrogen Bonding, Hydrophobic Interactions, HIV-1 Protease Assay, Radical Cyclisation, X-ray Crystallography.

INTRODUCTION

Human Immunodeficiency virus (HIV-1) is the causative agent of the acquired immunodeficiency syndrome (AIDS). Approximately 36.9 million people around the world are living with HIV-1/AIDS infection at the end of 2017, according to WHO (World Health Organization) and UNAIDS (The Joint United Nations Program on HIV-1/AIDS) [1]. However, there has been a decline in the number of HIV-1 infections each year due to the discovery of many drugs that halt the viral replication at various stages in the HIV-1 life cycle. Fixed dose combination of various classes of drugs as a part of highly active antiretroviral therapy (HAART) has proven to be successful in managing HIV-1/AIDS infections around the world.

HIV-1 is a highly mutable retrovirus infecting white blood cells, CD4$^+$ T-lymphocytes, which are critical to the immune system. Attack of the virus weakens the individuals' immune system and renders them susceptible to life-threatening opportunistic infections such as pneumonia, tuberculosis, herpes, tumors, *etc*. Different targets for the drugs in the HIV-1 life cycle are shown in Fig. (**1**). In this chapter, we will provide a brief summary of the various classes of drugs, however, our focus will be on the discovery of HIV-1 protease inhibitors, including work from our own laboratory.

HIV-1 replicates inside the host cell to produce DNA from its RNA, hence referred to as retrovirus. The first stage in the viruses' life cycle is the infection of a suitable host cell such as a CD4+ T-lymphocyte. Entry of HIV-1 into the host cell requires the presence of certain receptors on the cell surface such as CD4 receptors and co-receptors such as CCR5 or CXCR4. These receptors interact with HIV-1's three surface group (gp120) glycoproteins that are non-covalently associated with three transmembrane (gp41) protein subunits. The gp120-gp41 complex undergoes further conformational changes allowing the fusion peptide sequence to enter into the host cell and facilitate the cell fusion. Drugs capable of inhibiting this step are called entry/fusion inhibitors, which act on the outside of the host cell and offer potential advantage of lacking cross resistance to currently available therapeutics [2].

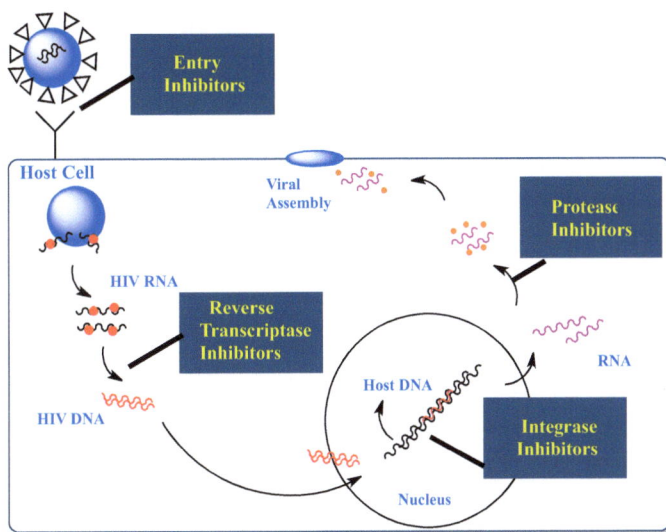

Fig. (1). The HIV-1 life cycle and potential targets for antiviral drugs.

The result of viral and cell membrane fusion allows the viral capsid to enter the host cell cytoplasm. Viral RNA is then released from the capsid and the first viral enzyme, reverse transcriptase (RT), transcribes single-stranded viral RNA to double-stranded DNA, called proviral DNA. Drugs that interfere in this process are called reverse transcriptase inhibitors (RTIs) and include the nucleoside and non-nucleoside RTIs. Azidothymidine (AZT) was the first anti-HIV-1 drug developed in this class.

In the next step of viral replication, the pro-viral DNA is inserted into the host cell genome using the second viral enzyme, HIV-1 integrase. After the integration of the viral DNA into the host cell, multiple copies of viral m-RNA are produced which are then transported from nucleus into the cytoplasm. Next step is the translation of the viral m-RNA in the cytoplasm to produce viral proteins. Viral core proteins are produced as long polypeptide chains that must be cleaved into smaller polypeptides in order to become functional. This is facilitated by the third viral enzyme, HIV-1 protease. The cleavage of the viral core proteins into functional proteins is essential for the survival and maturation of the virus. Hence the protease enzyme is considered to be a key target for the discovery of antiretroviral drugs known as protease inhibitors. Functional viral proteins and viral m-RNA then assemble at cell membrane and new virions released by a process called viral budding, and ready to infect new healthy host cells.

Currently, the following 5 Classes of HIV-1 drugs have been approved:

I. Entry inhibitors/Fusion inhibitors – *e.g.* enfuvirtide, maraviroc
II. Nucleoside reverse transcriptase inhibitors (NTRIs or "nukes") – *e.g.* retrovir (AZT), abacavir, lamivudine, emtricitabine
III. Non- nucleoside reverse transcriptase inhibitors (NNTRIs or "non-nukes") – *e.g.* efavirenz, nevirapine, etravirine, rilpivirine
IV. Integrase inhibitors – *e.g.* raltegravir
V. Protease inhibitors – *e.g.* indinavir, saquinavir, ritonavir, amprenavir, tipranavir, darunavir

Entry Inhibitors

To date only two entry inhibitors, maraviroc (selzentry) and enfuvirtide (fuzion) have received FDA approval and are available in the clinic. These inhibitors act by preventing the fusion of the HIV-1 with the host cell membrane either by mimicking the natural protein substrate or by interacting with the receptors involved in this process. Maraviroc is an orally-active small molecule that targets the co-receptor CCR5 and enfuvirtide is an injectable peptidic drug.

Enfuvirtide [3] is a membrane fusion inhibitor and is a 36-amino acid polypeptide (Ac-Tyr-Thr-Ser-Leu-Ile-His-Ser-Leu-Ile-Glu-Glu-Ser-Gln-Asn-Gln-Gln-Glu-Lys-Asn-Glu-Gln-Glu-Leu-Leu-Glu-Leu-Asp-Lys-Trp-Ala-Ser-Leu-Trp-Asn-Trp-Phe-NH$_2$). This linear synthetic peptide Fig. (**2**) was designed based on the structure of the HIV-1 fusion glycoprotein gp41. It is used in combination with other antiretroviral agents, for the treatment of HIV-1-infected individuals and AIDS patients. The development of cross resistance to this class of drugs is rare as it interferes in the earlier stage of viral entry. Enfuvirtide is synthesized using solid phase synthesis of three main fragments, followed by solution phase condensation of the fragments and purification of the deprotected crude enfuvirtide by chromatography [4]. As enfuvirtide is a peptide and not orally absorbed it is used in the clinic as an injectable and administered by subcutaneous route.

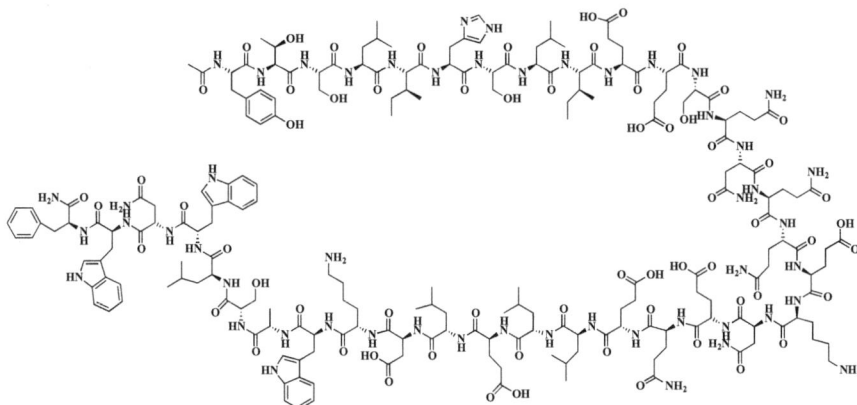

Fig. (2). Structure of enfuvirtide.

Enfuvirtide disrupts viral entry by competitively binding to the HIV-1 transmembrane protein gp41, thus inhibiting the formation of gp120-gp41complex which aids in cell fusion. The co-receptor CCR5 is a chemokine receptor found primarily in cells of the immune system and its inhibition by Maraviroc Fig. (**3**) [5] has proven to be an attractive anti-retroviral therapy.

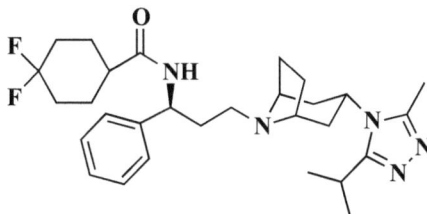

Fig. (3). Structure of maraviroc.

Synthesis of maraviroc [6] by Pfizer is shown in (Scheme **1**). It involves reductive amination of the aldehyde **1** with amine **2** to give the intermediate **3**. This is followed by deprotection of the t-boc group to furnish compound **4**. Coupling of compound **4** with 4,4-difluorocyclohexanecarboxylic acid (**5**) gave the desired final product, maraviroc.

Nucleoside Reverse Transcriptase Inhibitors (NRTIs)

Zidovudine (AZT) [7] was the first approved HIV-1/AIDS drug. It is a nucleoside analog or 'nuke' which works by inhibiting the viral reverse transcriptase enzyme. AZT gets incorporated in the growing viral DNA strand and since it has an azido group on the ribose instead of hydroxy, the elongation of the chain cannot occur resulting in blockage of DNA synthesis. HIV-1 reverse transcriptase enzyme is a heterodimer consisting of two subunits p66 and p51. The p66 subunit is responsible for the activity of the enzyme whereas p51 subunit is believed to play a structural role. NRTI's bind to the active site of the p66 subunit and prevent the reverse transcription of the viral RNA.

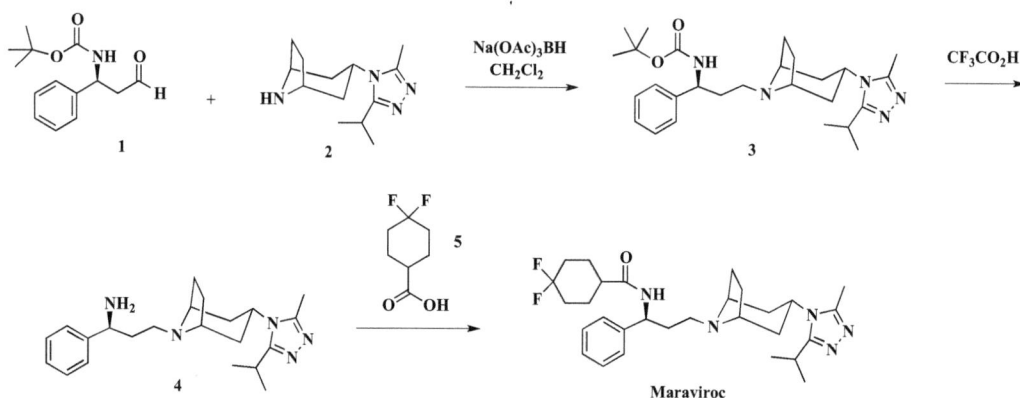

Scheme 1. Synthesis of maraviroc.

AZT is used as a key component in HAART therapy. It was approved by FDA in 1987 and subsequently being used extensively in the clinic. It has also been used to reduce the probability of transmission of the disease from infected mothers to the newly born children.

Synthesis of AZT from thymidine is shown in (Scheme **2**). The key step is the conversion of thymidine (**6**) to 2,3′-anhydro-5′-*O*-(4-methoxybenzoyl)-thymidine (**7**). Further ring opening of **7** with lithium azide followed by 5′-*O*-deprotection afforded AZT in 73% overall yield [8].

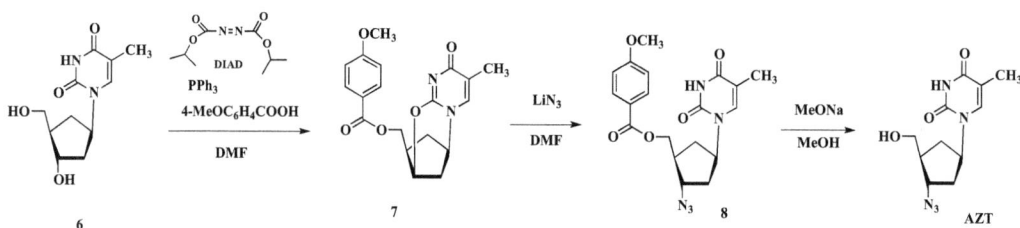

Scheme 2. Synthesis of AZT.

Abacavir is a carbocyclic nucleoside analog which is also used in the clinic as a HIV-1 reverse transcriptase inhibitor. Abacavir was synthesized by coupling of two key intermediates **13** and **14** followed by hydrolysis of the acetyl group (Scheme **3**) [9].

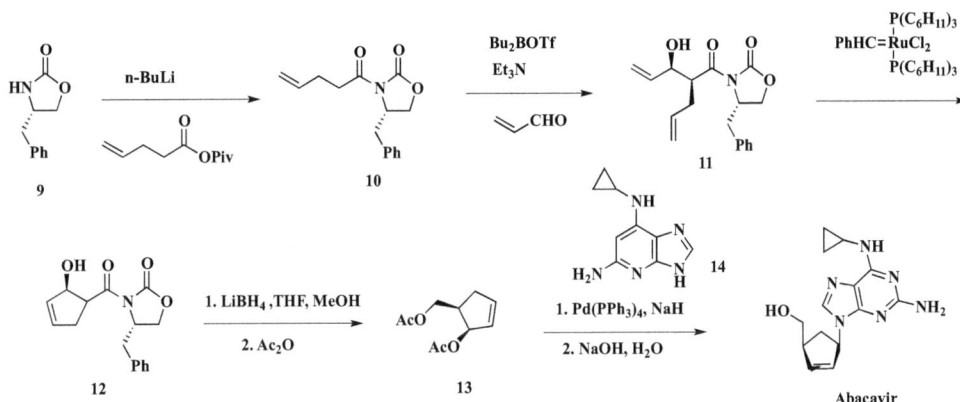

Scheme 3. Synthesis of abacavir.

Non-Nucleoside Reverse Transcriptase Inhibitors (NNRTIs)

Although NRTIs have been widely used in the clinic, there were also concerns about the selectivity and the side effects of this class of drugs. In addition, HIV-1 developing resistance to NRTIs have led to investigate NNRTIs with the aim to have activity against resistant organisms and demonstrate fewer side effects.

Unlike NRTIs, the NNRTIs bind to the allosteric hydrophobic pocket near the catalytic site of the p66 subunit and cause a conformation change in the reverse transcriptase enzyme preventing it from performing its normal function. The first generation of NNRTIs [10] were designed to fit in the hydrophobic pocket incorporating a tricyclic ring system. The two aromatic rings of NNRTIs such as nevirapine assumed to resemble the wings of the butterfly and the hydrophilic center as the body. Second generation NNRTIs such as etravirine (intelence) have a diaryl pyrimidine ring and known to exist in different conformations resulting in stronger binding interactions with the enzyme and improved activity against mutant strains of HIV-1 (Fig. **4**).

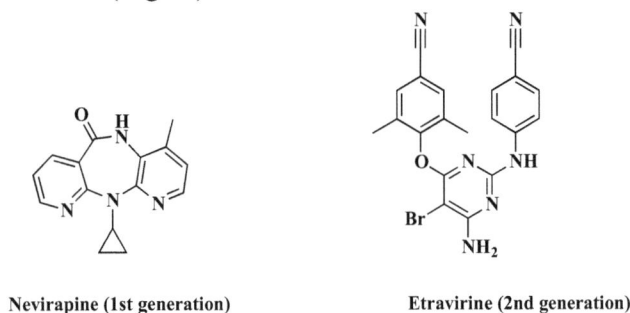

Nevirapine (1st generation)   **Etravirine (2nd generation)**

Fig. (4). Examples of NNRTIs.

Nevirapine is the first NNRTI approved by the FDA in 1996. It is synthesized by the condensation of 3-amino-2-chloro-4-methyl pyridine (**15**) with 2-chloronicotinyl chloride (**16**) to yield the 2,2'-dihaloamide **17**. In the next step displacement of the 2'-chlorine atom by amino cyclopropane yielded the desired amine **18**. Ring closure of the dipyridodiazepinone **18** was affected by heating the dianion generated by sodium hydride to yield nevirapine (Scheme **4**) [11].

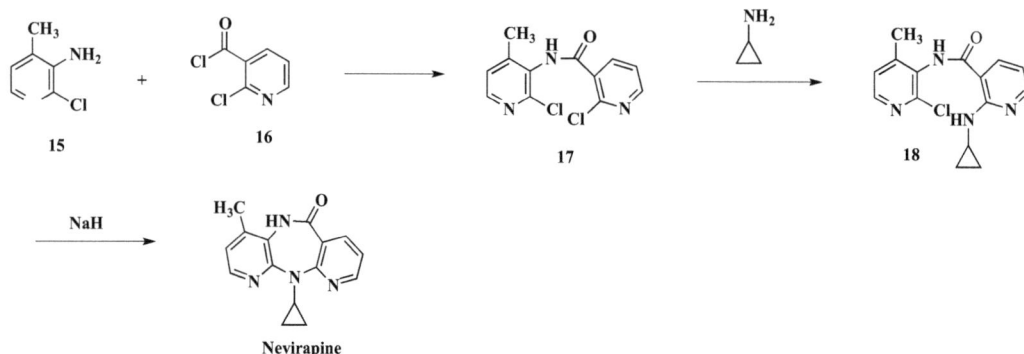

Scheme 4. Synthesis of nevirapine.

The diaryl pyrimidine based NNRTs constitute the second generation drugs and have been successfully used in the clinic against mutant viruses. Etravirine (TMC-125) is an example of the drug in this class which was approved by FDA in 2008 along with other antiretroviral agents for use in adult patients with multi-drug resistant HIV-1 infections. Synthesis of etravirine [12] is shown in (Scheme **5**).

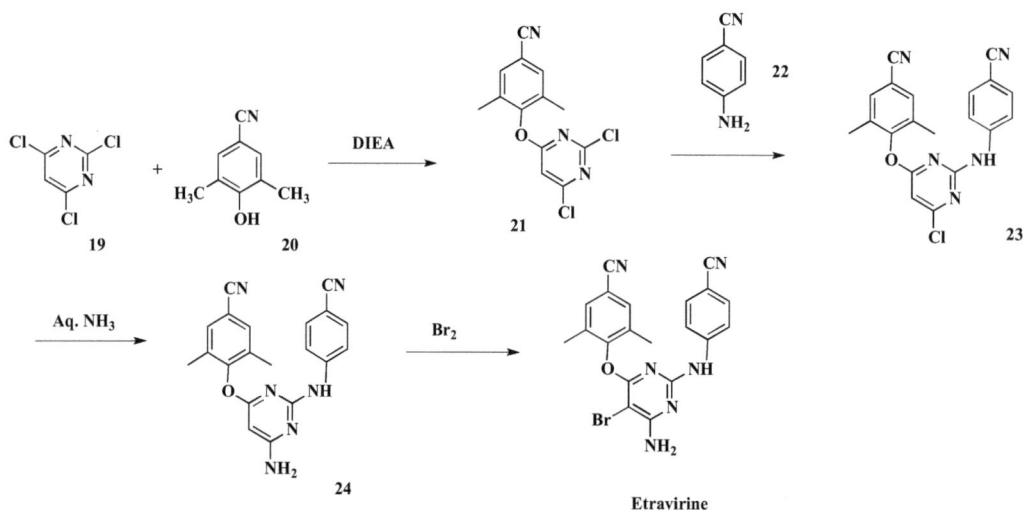

Scheme 5. Synthesis of etravirine.

The synthesis involves nucleophilic substitution of chlorine in the trihalo compound **19** with phenol derivative **20** to yield compound **21** which when treated with 4-cyano aniline (**22**) gave compound **23**. Aminolysis of **23** yielded **24** which on bromination gave the desired product etravirine.

Integrase Inhibitors

Integrase [13] is a viral enzyme responsible for the insertion of the viral genome into the DNA of the host cell. This integration is a key step in the replication of the virus and blocking this step will stop the multiplication of the virus. Integrase inhibitors (*e.g.* raltegravir, Fig. (**5**)) have become part of HAART regimen and are widely used in the clinic to halt viral replication. Synthesis of raltegravir [14] is shown below (Scheme **6**).

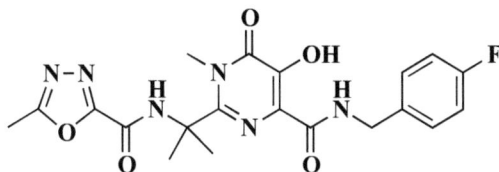

Fig. (5). Structure of raltegravir (isentress)

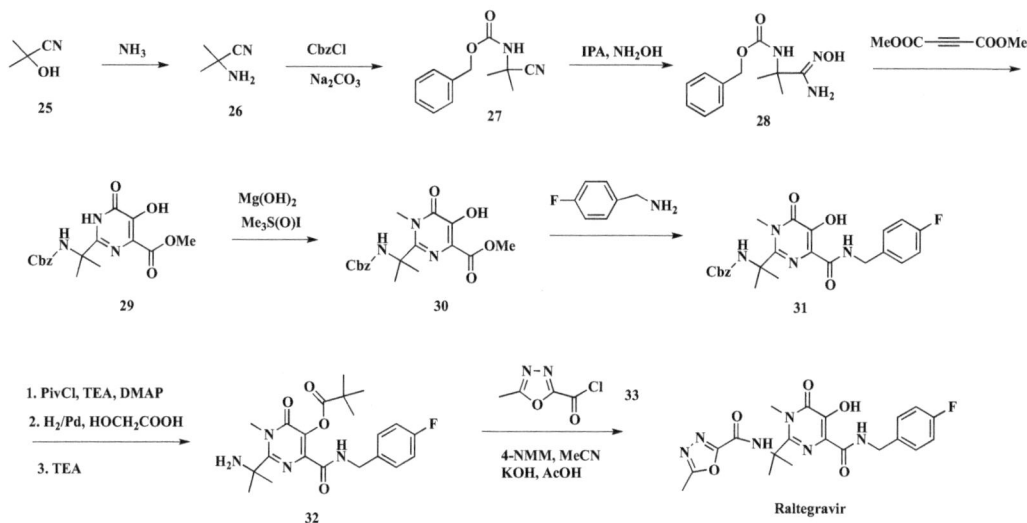

Scheme 6. Synthesis of raltegravir.

Treatment of compound **25** with ammonia gave the amine **26**. Protection of the amino group in **26** followed by reaction with hydroxylamine yielded compound **28**. Compound **28** was further treated with dialkyl acetylene dicarboxylate to give compound **29**. N-alkylation of compound **29** with trimethylsulfoxonium iodide gave **30**, which upon treatment with p-fluorobenzyl amine produced compound **31**. Compound **31** was converted to **32**, which on treatment with the acid chloride **33** yielded raltegravir.

HIV-1 Protease Inhibitors-Structure Based Drug Design

The discovery of HIV-1 protease inhibitors represents the classic example of structure-based drug design [15]. The X-ray crystal structure of HIV-1 protease was determined in 1989 and several inhibitors were soon developed based on the knowledge of the configuration of the active site. Protease inhibitors were designed to mimic the transition state of the cleavage of the protease's substrates. HIV-1 protease inhibitors fit the active site of the HIV-1 aspartic protease and were rationally designed utilizing knowledge of the aspartyl protease's mode of action. The most promising transition state mimic was hydroxyethylamine, which led to the discovery of the first protease inhibitor, saquinavir. Following that discovery, other HIV-1 protease inhibitors were designed using the same principle.

Binding Site

HIV-1 protease belongs to a family of aspartic acid proteases and exists as a homodimer of two 99 amino acid containing proteins. The folding of the identical proteins leads to a C2 symmetric tertiary structure. Each monomer contributes an aspartic acid residue that is essential for catalysis, Asp-25 and Asp-25´. Key features of the active site include four hydrophobic binding pockets (S_1, S_2, $S_1^{'}$, and $S_2^{'}$) and hydrogen bond donors necessary for tight binding to the substrate. Ile50 and Ile50' play an important role in hydrogen bonding with a structural water molecule. The water molecule is important in increasing the affinity between enzyme and substrate. HIV-1 proteases catalyze the hydrolysis of peptide bonds of the substrate with high sequence selectivity and catalytic efficiency. The aspartyl residues are involved in the hydrolysis of the scissile peptide bonds. The preferred cleavage site for this enzyme is the N-terminal side of proline residues, especially between phenylalanine and proline or tyrosine and proline.

The HIV-1 protease inhibitors [16] in clinical use have all the structural features necessary for tight binding into the active site of the enzyme. They are designed to include hydrophobic substituents that are clearly necessary for tight fitting into the hydrophobic binding pockets. Additionally, a common feature to nearly all the protease inhibitors is the presence of a free hydroxyl group which plays an important role in hydrogen bonding directly with aspartic acid residues 25 and 25' in the active site. Another set of hydrogen bond acceptors allow hydrogen bonding to a conserved water molecule that is, in turn, hydrogen bonded to the isoleucine residues 50 and 50' of the protease backbone. Fig. (**6**) illustrates these bindings with a pictorial representation of the drug, indinavir as it fits into the active site of the HIV-1 protease.

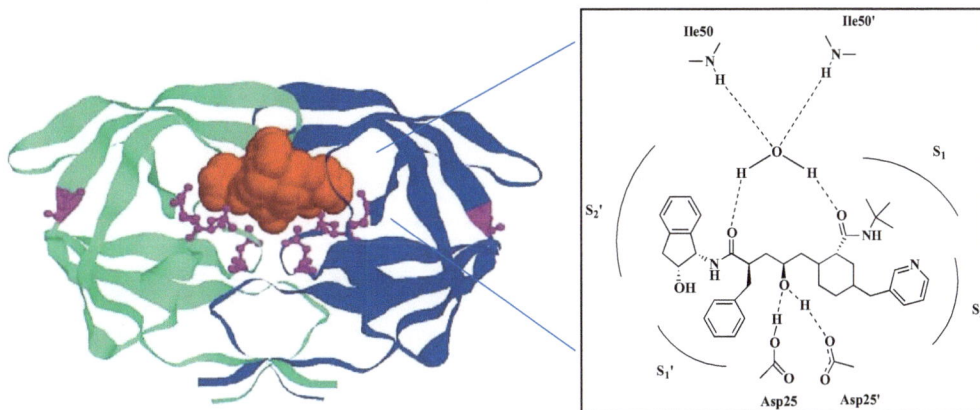

Fig. (6). X-ray crystal structure of HIV-1 protease bound to the inhibitor (Indinavir) (PDB code 2avo).

Since HIV-1 protease inhibitors were first introduced in 1995, they have greatly benefited those infected by HIV-1 by suppressing the virus and reducing mortality. As already pointed out HIV-1 protease is a viral encoded aspartyl enzyme which catalyzes the cleavage of a large precursor protein into an array of smaller and functional, viral proteins. Competitive inhibitors are used to bind to the protease and block its function, thereby suppressing the virus, which cannot transform to its mature, infectious form. Although HIV-1 protease is similar to mammalian aspartyl proteases like rennin in terms of its structure and function, however in the host there is virtually no cross-reactivity between the HIV-1 protease and normal human protease gene products. It is this lack of cross-reactivity that gives the protease inhibitors their outstanding safety profile. Some of the protease inhibitors approved by FDA for clinical use are shown in (Figs. **7** & **8**).

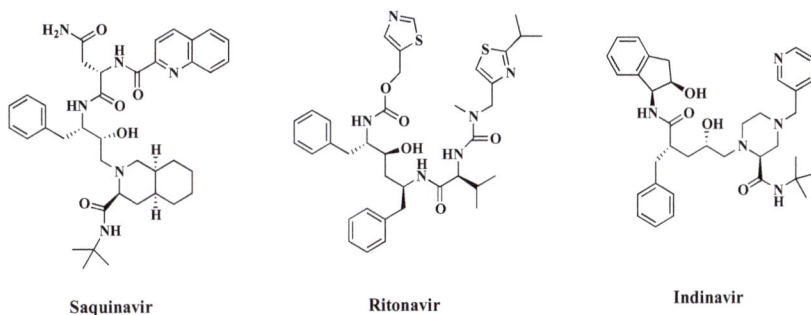

Saquinavir   Ritonavir   Indinavir

Fig. (7). First generation peptidomimetic HIV-1 protease inhibitors on the market.

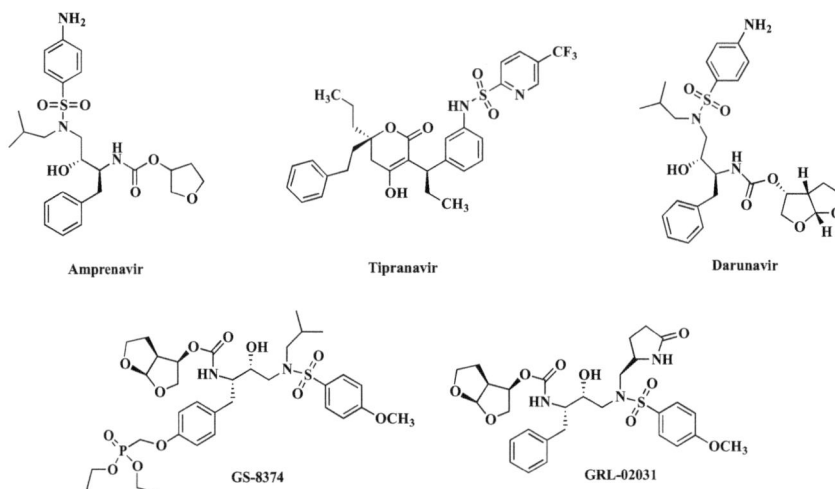

Fig. (8). Protease inhibitors containing sulfonamide functional moiety

Saquinavir was the first protease inhibitor that was approved and its incorporation in HAART has led to significant enhancement of HIV-1 management and improved quality of life in AIDS patients. After the discovery of saquinavir several other HIV-1 protease inhibitors were discovered such as ritonavir, indinavir, nelfinavir and lopinavir. Being peptidic in nature these drugs suffered from poor pharmacokinetic properties including showing low serum concentration after the drug administration and gastrointestinal side effects was also noted. In addition, the rapid emergence of multidrug resistant strains has highly compromised the HAART therapy. As the search for the newer protease inhibitors continued, compounds containing a sulfonamide group as the binding moiety in place of an amide group were discovered which improved the oral bioavailability. Subsequent modification of the end groups of these inhibitors resulted in stronger binding interactions with the protease backbone resulting in enhanced activity against resistant organisms. Examples of sulfonamide containing HIV-1 protease inhibitors include amprenavir, tipranvir, darunavir and investigational candidates GS8374 and GRL02031.

Towards the design of darunavir [17] the investigators primarily focused on reducing peptidic features, molecular weight and structural complexity of the earlier inhibitors. A number of nonpeptidic high-affinity for HIV-1 protease substrate were designed based on the 3D structures of protein ligand complex. Particularly the design of conformationally constrained molecules of cyclic ether template that could replace peptide bonds, retaining important binding interactions were explored. It was found that 3(*S*)-tetrahydrofuranyl urethane in the inhibitors showed enhanced potency which led to the development of amprenavir [18]. The tetrahydrofuranyl subunit is found in the structures of natural products such as monensin and various ginkgolides.

X-ray structures of 3(*S*)-tetrahydrofuranyl urethane-bearing inhibitors revealed weak hydrogen bonding between the tetrahydrofuranyl oxygen and the main chain aspartic acids (Asp-29 and Asp-30) as well as van der Waals interactions in the S2-site. Critical analysis of the saquinavir-bound protease X-ray crystal structure led to the discovery of a stereochemically defined bicyclic tetrahydrofuran (bis-THF) ligand that appeared to effectively hydrogen bond with both Asp-29 and Asp-30. Thus, inhibitors were synthesized with improved solubility, reduced peptidic features and low molecular weight compared to saquinavir. This led to the development of highly potent protease inhibitor, darunavir. Darunavir (TMC114) with a bis-THF as the P2 ligand and p-aminosulfonamide as the P2' ligand showed very impressive inhibitory properties. The X-ray crystal structure of darunavir-bound protease revealed that the bis-THF ring oxygens are involved in effective hydrogen bonding interactions with both the backbone NH's of Asp-29 and Asp-30 present in the S2 subsite. Clinical trials of the darunavir demonstrated significant reduction in the viral load when compared with the existing protease inhibitors. Synthesis of darunavir is presented in (Scheme **7**) [19].

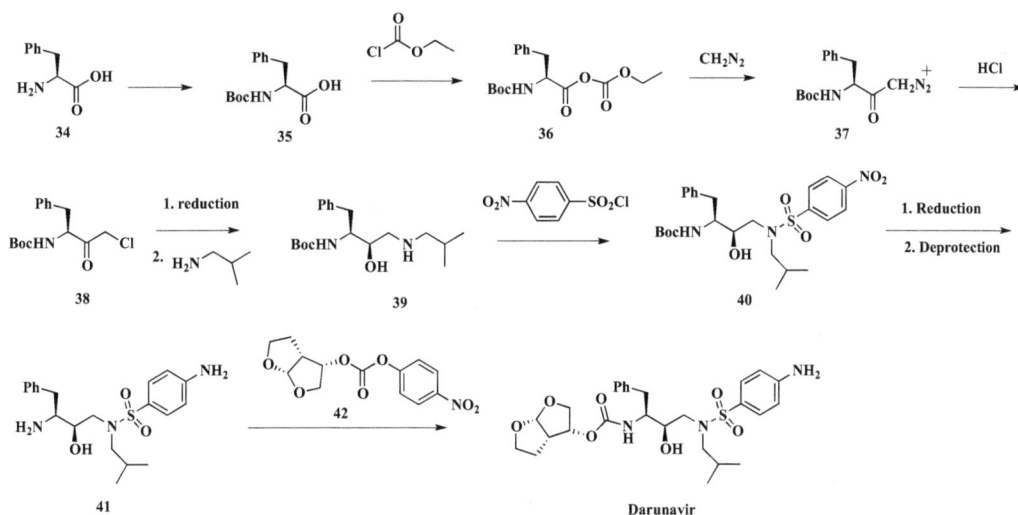

Scheme 7. Synthesis of darunavir.

Thus (*S*)-phenylalanine (**34**) is converted to compound **35** by protecting the amine. Treatment of compound **35** with ethylchloroformate gave **36**. Compound **36** was further treated with diazomethane, followed by hydrochloric acid to yield the alkyl halide **38**. Reduction of compound **38** followed by nucleophilic substitution with isobutyl amine gave compound **39**. Compound **39** was converted to compound **40** using p-nitrosulfonyl chloride. Reduction of the nitro group in **40** followed by deprotection of the t-boc group gave the amine **41**, which on further treatment with compound **42** yielded darunavir.

Analogs of darunavir incorporating hexahydrofuropyranol derived P2 ligands have retained potent activity against resistant HIV-1 organisms similar to that of darunavir [20]. Analysis of X-ray crystal structures of compound **43** (Fig. **9** bound with HIV-1 protease showed that the stereochemistry of the ligand and position of the oxygen are critical in binding to the HIV-1 protease enzyme. Furthermore, the extra methylene unit in the ligand maximizes the binding interactions with the hydrophobic pocket in the S2-site more effectively compared to the bis-THF in darunavir.

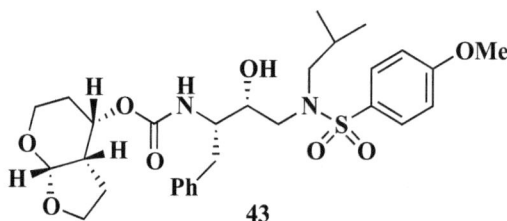

Fig. (9). Structure of 4-hexahydrofuropyranol-derived urethane derivative, **43**.

As noted above, sulfonamide derived HIV-1 protease inhibitors such as darunavir and analogs incorporate open chain conformationally flexible sulfonamide group in their structures.

We speculated that conformationally restricted cyclic sulfonamide HIV-1 protease inhibitors, represented by structure **44** Fig. (**10**) might offer advantages over open chain analogs by maximizing binding interactions with the backbone of the protease enzyme. To test the hypothesis, we synthesized a series of compounds related to **44** and determined their activities against HIV-1 protease enzyme [21]. General structures represented by **44** also offered an opportunity to explore biological activity associated with lipophilicity and stereochemistry of the crucially important R' functionality. We believe cyclic sulfonamides will serve as novel pharmacophore for the discovery of drugs involving other biological targets.

After our work was published, a macrocyclic sulfonamide inhibitor **45** [22] was synthesized and found to be highly active against HIV-1 protease. Inhibitor **45** Fig. (**11**) remained highly potent activity against resistant organisms. The flexible P1'-P2' macrocyclic packs between the S1'-S2' subsites in a zigzag crown-like shape. The high affinity of the inhibitor was attributed to the new water-mediated hydrogen bonding interactions of the macrocyclic ring oxygen with backbone atoms at the S2'-site.

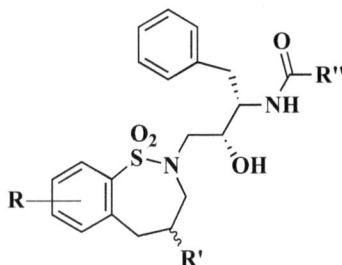

44

Fig. (10). Design of novel cyclic sulfonamide HIV-1 protease inhibitors

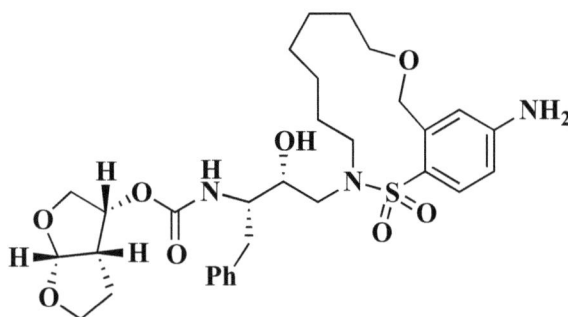

45

Fig. (11). Structure of the macrocyclic HIV-1 protease inhibitor, **45**.

Design of Novel Conformationally Restricted Sulfonamides

As pointed out above we were interested to discover novel pharmacophores which could be used in drug discovery.

Thus, we conceived and synthesized novel conformationally restricted sulfonamides and demonstrated that they possessed potent activities against HIV-1 protease which will be discussed in detail in this chapter.

Sulfonamides are well known for their diverse biological activities, and have been used as antibacterial, antitumor, diuretics, anticonvulsants and protease inhibitors. The importance of sulfonamide group for the HIV-1 protease inhibitory activity may be attributed to the binding to the HIV-1 protease involving, (i) strong hydrogen bonding with the structural water molecule at the active site, (ii) hydrophobic interactions of the phenyl group attached to the sulfonyl group with the S_2' of the enzyme and (iii) increased water solubility. It is important to note that most of the protease inhibitors described in the literature bearing sulfonamide functional group are all open chain compounds and therefore they are likely to assume many conformations. However, we speculated that by making cyclic sulfonamides we would be able to maximize binding interactions with the enzyme. To test the hypothesis, we incorporated cyclic sulfonamide pharmacophore in our HIV-1 protease inhibitors represented by the general structure **44**. The first synthesis of the novel seven membered cyclic sulfonamide ring was described from our laboratories involving radical reaction.

We have described synthesis of conformationally restricted sulfonamides [23] represented by formula **46** wherein the R' substituents are alkyl, aryl and aryl alkyl groups (Fig. **12**). The ring size could be six, seven or eight atoms. In this chapter, we wish to summarize the design and synthesis of compounds represented by the general structure **44** which have been found to be potent inhibitors of HIV-1 protease. Several HIV-1 protease inhibitor drugs shown in Figs. (**7**) & (**8**), have been successfully used in AIDS patients. In general, our compounds represent novel pharmacophores and are comparable in potency with the protease inhibitors used in the clinic. We hoped that by selectively modifying the structure of **44**, these novel compounds might show improvements in the spectrum of activity against resistant organisms and also show improvements in pharmacokinetic properties.

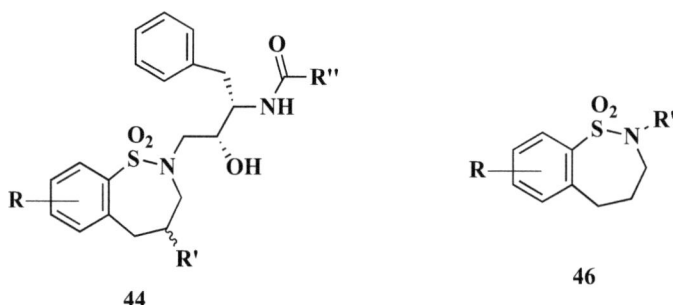

Fig. (12). Novel protease inhibitors – core structure containing sulfonamide.

As mentioned above compounds represented by structure **46** were synthesized using a radical cyclization process. Thus, treatment of compound **47**, with tributyltin hydride (TBTH) and azobisisobutyronitrile (AIBN) in refluxing toluene solution yielded **46** *via* **48** and **49** (Scheme **8**).

The above synthetic scheme has been extended for the synthesis of the corresponding N-H compound **53** (Scheme **9**). Treatment of 2-bromo benzene sulfonyl chloride (**50**) with allylamine (**51**) yielded the sulfonamide **52**. Radical reaction of **52** provided **53**. Treatment of **53** with the epoxide **54** furnished the compound **55**. Compound **55** showed K_i of 470 nM in HIV-1 protease assay. Compound **55** when converted to compound **57** was found to be inactive.

Compound **57** demonstrated the importance of the presence of the hydroxy group and binding interactions with the carbonyl group of the open chain carbamate residue for antiviral activity.

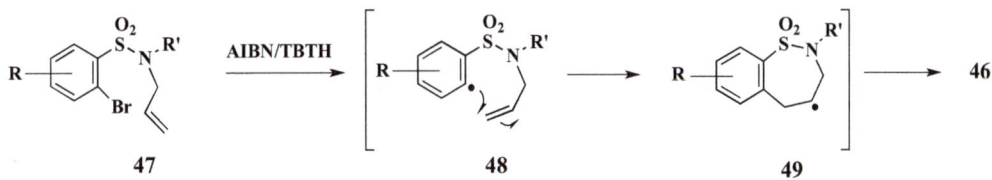

R' = Alkyl, aryl or aryl alkyl groups

Scheme 8. Synthesis of 7-membered cyclic sulfonamide using radical cyclization.

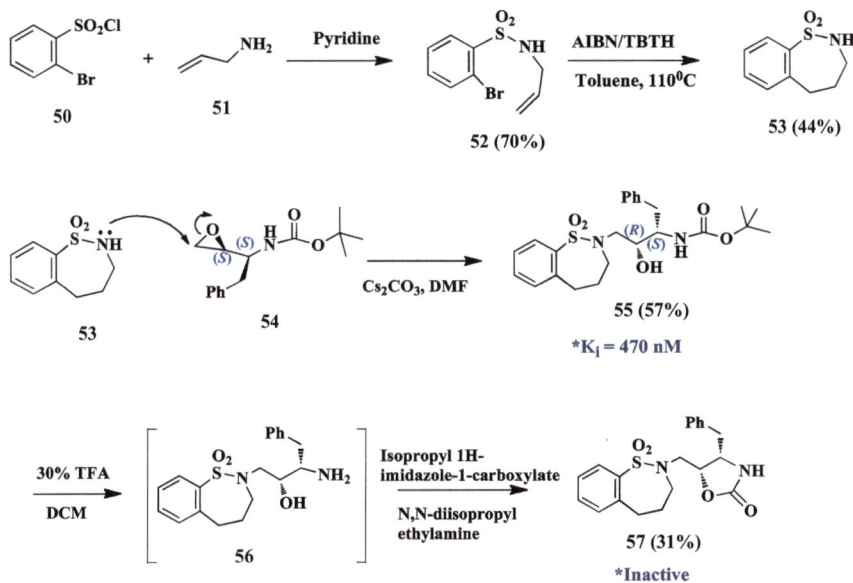

Scheme 9. Synthesis of novel HIV-1 protease inhibitor **55**.

Using similar approach, we synthesized compounds **53a-e** from **52a-e**, respectively (Scheme **10**). This allowed us to synthesize compounds represented by structure **44** by derivatization of the free –NH- function.

Based on molecular modeling we considered to introduce a methyl group at C4 on the sulfonamide ring. The synthesis of C4-methyl cyclic sulfonamide is shown (Scheme **11**). Radical cyclisation of **52a** yielded racemate **53a**. Treatment of **53a** with the epoxide **54** yielded **58** as a mixture of diastereoisomers, which could not be separated. Removal of the t-boc furnished the amine. At this stage we were able to separate the two diastereoisomers **59** and **60**. X-ray crystallographic analysis of **59** established its absolute stereochemistry as $4R, 2'R, 3'S$ Fig. (**13**) and therefore the absolute configuration of **60** will be $4S, 2'R, 3'S$. Compounds **59** and **60** were then converted to the t-boc derivatives **61** and **62** respectively. In HIV-1 protease assay **62** with K_i value of 29 nM was considerably more potent than **61**, which showed a K_i value of 1000 nm. This dramatic difference in protease inhibitory activities of **61** ($4R,2'R,3'S$) and **62** ($4S,2'R,3'S$) suggested the importance of stereochemistry at C4 to be (S) for optimum HIV-1 protease inhibitory activity.

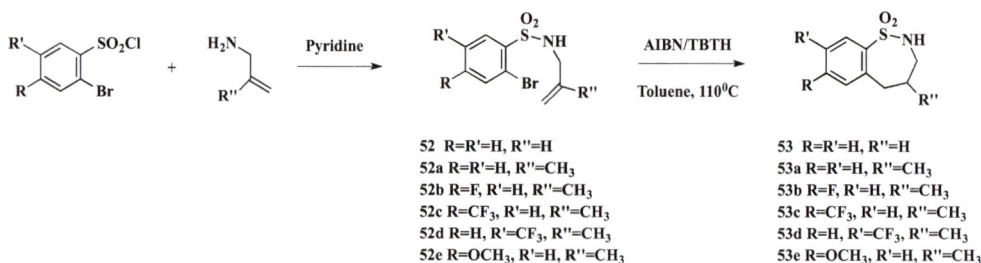

52 R=R'=H, R''=H
52a R=R'=H, R''=CH$_3$
52b R=F, R'=H, R''=CH$_3$
52c R=CF$_3$, R'=H, R''=CH$_3$
52d R=H, R'=CF$_3$, R''=CH$_3$
52e R=OCH$_3$, R'=H, R''=CH$_3$

53 R=R'=H, R''=H
53a R=R'=H, R''=CH$_3$
53b R=F, R'=H, R''=CH$_3$
53c R=CF$_3$, R'=H, R''=CH$_3$
53d R=H, R'=CF$_3$, R''=CH$_3$
53e R=OCH$_3$, R'=H, R''=CH$_3$

Scheme 10. Synthesis of cyclic sulfonamides **53a-e**.

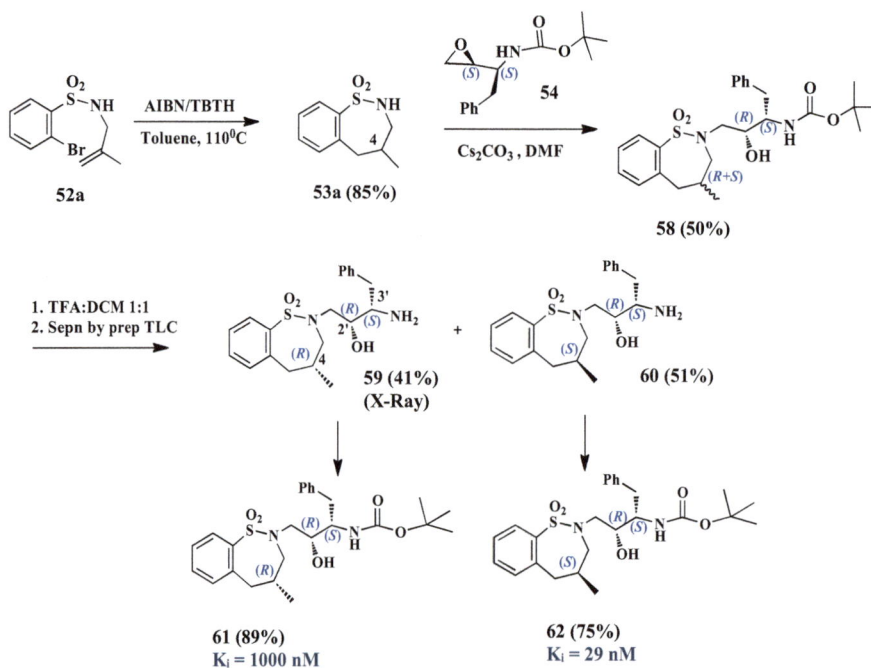

52a

53a (85%)

58 (50%)

1. TFA:DCM 1:1
2. Sepn by prep TLC

59 (41%)
(X-Ray)

60 (51%)

61 (89%)
K_i = 1000 nM

62 (75%)
K_i = 29 nM

Scheme 11. Synthesis of C4 methyl analogs.

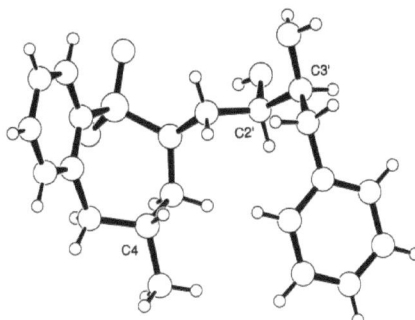

Fig. (13). X-ray crystallographic structure of compound **59**.

As 4*S* methyl group is important for optimal potency, we included the methyl group in our core structure and decided to study the effect of various N-substitutions. Thus, we made compounds **63-69** and their diastereoisomers. The C4(*R*) diastereoisomers, which are not shown here, were also analyzed in the protease assay and found to be inactive. Improved activity of **66** and **69** demonstrated that substitution at R1 is important for potency and possibly in preventing metabolism (Table **1**). The key interactions of the free hydroxyl group at 2' and the hydrogen bonding ability of the sulfonamide and the carbamate residues remain intact. Although **66** and **69** have nearly equal potency we preferred to have fluorine in our structures for further optimization studies because it is metabolically more stable than methoxy group in **69**.

This demonstrated that not only methyl group is important in improving the potency but it must also have the correct stereochemistry. We were later able to show by molecular modeling, the difference in the potency of the two diastereoisomers was due to differences in the binding interactions with the protease enzyme.

To investigate whether the carbamates in this series of compounds could be replaced by amides we made compound **70** which when tested in HIV-1 protease assay had a K_i value of 30 nM (Fig. **14**).

The X-ray crystallographic structure of compound **66** bound to the HIV-1 protease Fig. (**15**) was solved and was very informative. It was observed that compound **66** occupies the active site cavity of the protease and makes hydrogen bonding to the catalytic aspartic acid residues Asp25 and Asp25' through the hydroxyl group. The sulfonamide and the carbamate carbonyl form hydrogen bonds with a structural water molecule, which in turn hydrogen bonds with Ile 50 and Ile 50' of the protease (Fig. **16**).

Table 1. SAR of Novel HIV-1 protease inhibitors.

Compd No.	Substitution	K_i (nM)
63	$R_1 = R_2 = H$; $R_3 = $ Allyl	27
64	$R_1 = R_2 = H$; $R_3 = $ Et	34
65	$R_1 = R_2 = H$; $R_3 = $ Ph	350
66	$R_1 = F$; $R_2 = H$; $R_3 = $ t-butyl	20
67	$R_1 = CF_3$; $R_2 = H$; $R_3 = $ t-butyl	186
68	$R_1 = H$; $R_2 = CF_3$; $R_3 = $ t-butyl	100
69	$R_1 = OCH_3$; $R_2 = H$; $R_3 = $ t-butyl	19

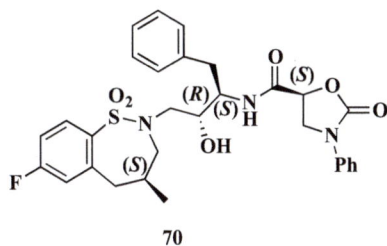

70

Fig. (14). Structure of the amide inhibitor.

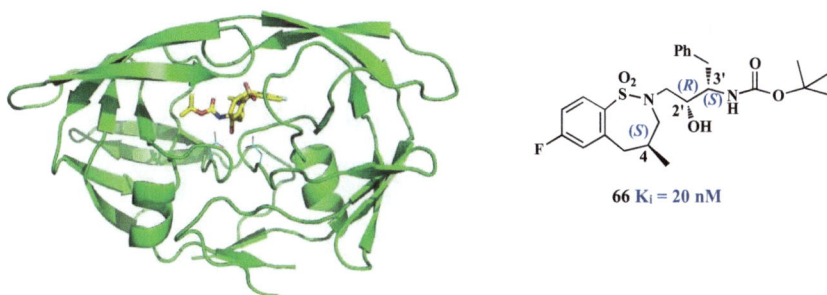

66 $K_I = 20$ nM

Fig. (15). X-ray crystallographic structure of compound **66** bound to HIV-1 protease enzyme (PDB code 3TH9).

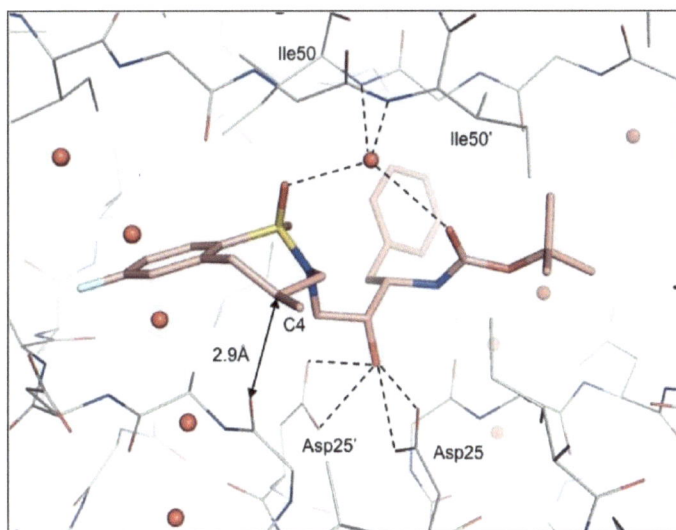

Fig. (16). X-ray crystallographic structure of compound **66** showing key interactions with the HIV-1 protease enzyme (PDB code 3TH9)

In addition to these favorable hydrogen bonding stabilization effects, C4-Me group of compound **66** has extensive hydrophobic interactions with side chains of Leu23, Val82, and Ile84.

When superimposed the X-ray structure of **66** with that of darunavir, a similar acyclic inhibitor, there is a nice overlay with exception of the aromatic sulfonamide plane, which is rotated by 42 degrees (Fig. **17**). The cyclizing linker, including C4, bridges towards the hydrophobic area of the active site occupied by the iso-butyl group of darunavir.

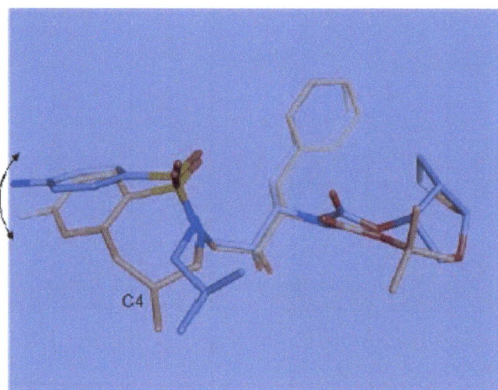

Fig. (17). Overlay of **66** with darunavir (PDB code 2hs1). Rotation of cyclized fluoro-phenyl with respect to non-cyclized aromatic plane is shown with arrow.

A B

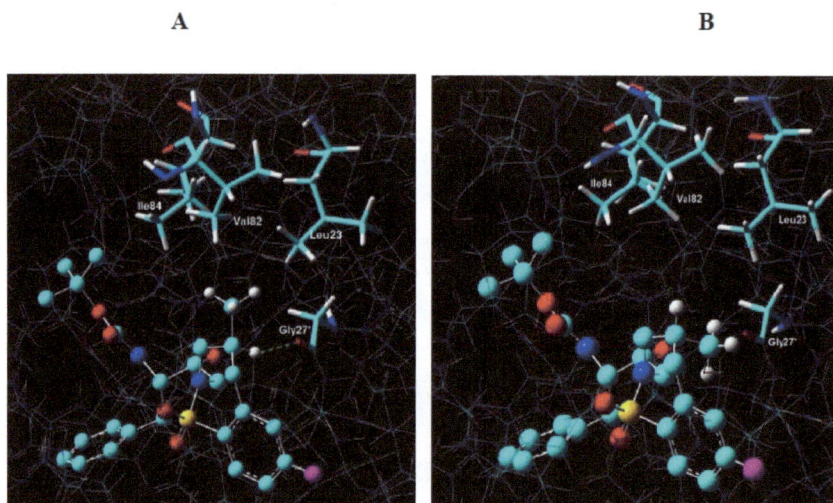

Fig. (18). (A) Molecular docking of compound **66** showing interactions of the C4(S) methyl group with the hydrophobic pocket. (B) Molecular docking of compound **66** with C4(R) methyl group showing no interactions with the hydrophobic pocket.

Furthermore, analyzing the X-ray crystallographic structure of compounds **66** bound with HIV-1 protease we found that the C4-Me (S configuration) in compound **66** is 2.9 angstroms away from the carbonyl oxygen of Gly27' (Fig. **18**). If the C4-Me configuration is changed to (R) instead of (S), an unfavorable repulsion would be created betwee18 the C4-Me and the Gly27' carbonyl group and the interactions to the hydrophobic pocket would be lost. These results support the experimental observation that compounds with the C4-methyl group in the (*S*) configuration possess optimum activity.

The X-ray crystallographic analysis of compound **66** also suggested that C4-Me group could be further extended in order to maximize the interactions with the hydrophobic pocket, thus enhancing potency. Hence, we decided to study the effect of various alkyl groups on the cyclic sulfonamide ring for their activities against HIV-1 protease. In addition, the molecular modeling suggested that the tetrahydrofuran carbamates similar to amprenavir and different than darunavir would provide stronger binding to the protease backbone through hydrogen bonding of Asp 29' and Asp30'. Thus, we synthesized compounds represented by the structure **71** incorporating all the above ideas. (Fig. **19**).

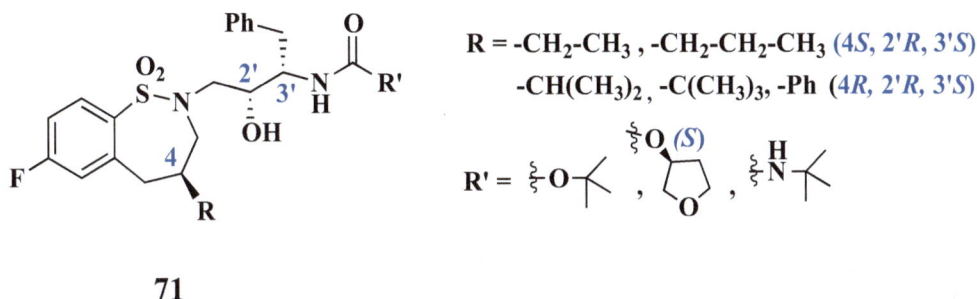

$R = $ -CH$_2$-CH$_3$, -CH$_2$-CH$_2$-CH$_3$ (4*S*, 2'*R*, 3'*S*)
    -CH(CH$_3$)$_2$, -C(CH$_3$)$_3$, -Ph (4*R*, 2'*R*, 3'*S*)

71

Fig. (19). Design of novel analogs based on the X-ray crystallographic analysis.

In order to synthesize C4 substituted analogs we had to modify the synthetic scheme as the substituted allyl amines were not commercially available. The results are summarized in (Scheme **12**). Thus, the treatment of 2-bromo-4 fluoro benzenesulfonyl chloride with 4-methoxybenzylamine gave the sulfonamide **72**. Reaction of compound **72** with substituted allyl bromides **73-76** in the presence of cesium carbonate and sodium iodide gave compounds **77-80** respectively. The synthesis of bromo compounds **73-76** is also shown. Deprotection of the p-methoxybenzyl group yielded compounds **81-84**. Radical cyclisation using AIBN and TBTH furnished the desired cyclic sulfonamides **85-88 in** excellent yields.

We also decided to make the C4-phenyl substitution and compare its activity with the alkyl substitution. The synthesis of the cyclic sulfonamide **91** with C4-Ph is shown below (Scheme **13**).

The –NH compounds **85-88** and **91** were then used to make the novel HIV-1 protease inhibitors (Scheme **14**). Treatment of –NH compounds with the commercially available chiral epoxide **54** in the presence of cesium carbonate and DMF yielded mixtures of diastereoisomers **92-96** respectively, which could not be separated. The mixture of diastereoismers could be separated when converted to corresponding amines by treatment with TFA. Hence, we obtained separated diastereoisomeric amines **97** and **102** from compound **92**. Similarly, other diastereoisomers were separated as shown in (Scheme **14**). We have previously established the absolute configuration in the C4-Me (*S*) diastereoisomer series by X-ray crystallography of the corresponding amine and corroborated further by X-ray crystal structure of compound **66** bound to the protease. The more polar (6% methanol in chloroform) diastereoisomers **102-104** were treated with di-tert-butyl dicarbonate and diisopropyl ethylamine to give the final products **107-109** respectively which showed potent activity as HIV-1 protease inhibitors. The corresponding derivatives obtained from the less polar diastereoisomers **97,** and **98** were found to be inactive and not reported in the paper. Treatment of the diastereoisomers **104-106** respectively with (*S*)-2,5-dioxopyrrolidin-1-yl (tetrahydrofuran-3-yl) carbonate (**110**) [24] and triethylamine in dichloromethane yielded **111-113**. The urea derivative **114** was synthesized by the treatment of **104** with tert-butyl isocyanate in the presence of magnesium bromide using 1,4-dioxane as solvent. Although the less polar diastereisomers were inactive in previous cases, compounds **99** and **100**, when converted into their tetrahydrofuran carbamates, **115** and **116** respectively, were found to be active. We have found that every case studied, it is the more polar diastereoisomeric amines when converted to the carbamates show activity.

The results of HIV-1 protease inhibitory assay of compounds **107-109** and **111-116** are summarized in Table (**2**). It was found that compounds with alkyl substitution were more potent than the aryl substitution. Compound **107** with C4-Et (*S*) on the cyclic sulfonamide ring was found to have the K_i value of 11 nM, which was a slight improvement in potency when compared with C4-Me (*S*) substitution as in compound **66** (K_i = 20 nM). C4-Pr (*S*) compound **108** had the K_i value of 28 nM. With the introduction of C4-iPr (*R*) group in compound **109** there was nearly 6-fold increase in the potency with K_i of 2.8 nM when compared to compound **66**. The urea derivative **114** was also found to be active with a K_i of 6.4 nM. However, when we made the C4-Ph analog **113** with a tetrahydrofuran carbamate, the potency was reduced with a K_i value of 34 nM. The introduction of tetrahydrofuran carbamate helped significantly improve the activity in compound **111** with a K_i of 360 pM. In the compound **112** with a C4-t-butyl (*R*) group there was further increase in activity when compared with compound **111**. In our series of cyclic sulfonamides compound **112** is the most potent analog with a K_i of 260 pM.

We have observed in previous cases where the C4 substitution was methyl, ethyl, or propyl that the diastereoisomers with C4(R) stereochemistry were inactive. However, when the diasteroisomers **115** and **116** were tested, we were surprised to find that they were active with a K_i value of 19 nM and 14 nM respectively. Although the diastereoisomers **115** and **116** were less active than **111** and **112** respectively, their potency could be explained by the X-ray crystallographic analysis. Compounds **112** and **116** when bound to the HIV-1 protease unequivocally demonstrated that both these compounds bind to the same hydrophobic pocket as the C4-Me (S) diastereoisomer and have similar interactions involving Asp25, Asp25', Ile 50 and Ile 50'. X-ray results also demonstrated that **112** and **116** assume different conformations of the seven membered sulfonamide rings (Fig. **22**). The same explanation we believe holds good for **111** and **115**. Although the inactive C4-Me (R) diastereoisomer could not be soaked into HIV protease apo crystals, molecular modeling suggests that the methyl group in this case was pushed away from the important hydrophobic binding site. The above X-ray crystallography results also confirmed the absolute stereochemistry of **111**, **112**, **115** and **116**. Perhaps it should also be noted that the absolute stereochemistry at C2' and C3'were derived from the absolute stereochemistry of the epoxide **54** and the remaining asymmetric center was defined from compound **110** used in the preparation of the carbamate.

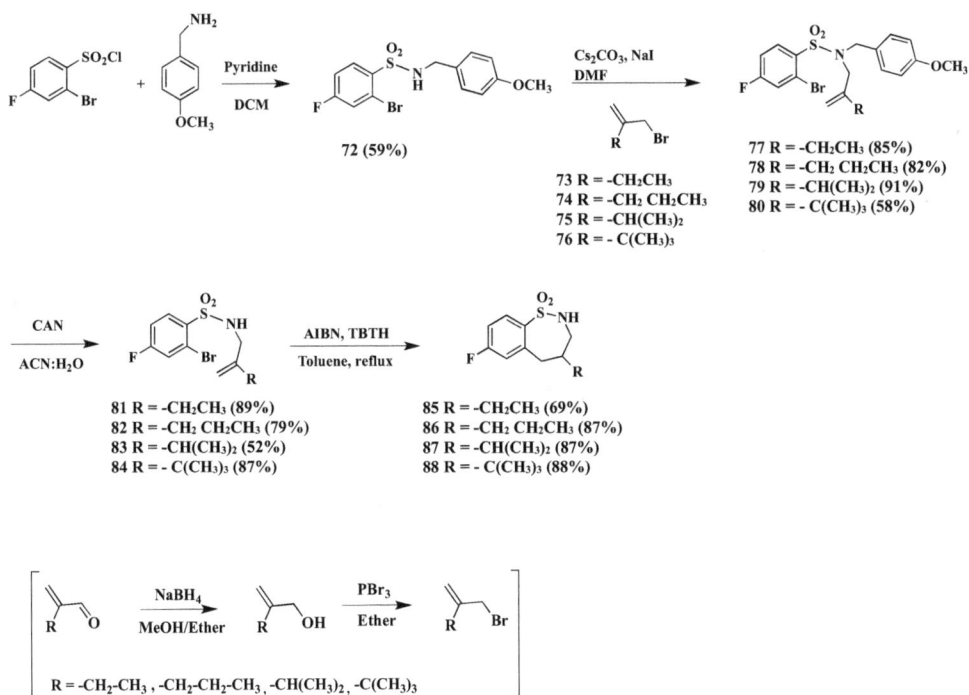

Scheme 12. Synthesis of novel C4 substituted analogs.

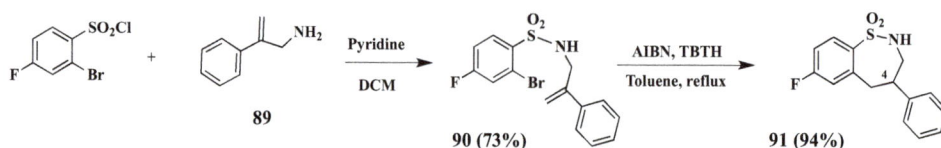

Scheme 13. Synthesis of C4-phenyl sulfonamide **91**.

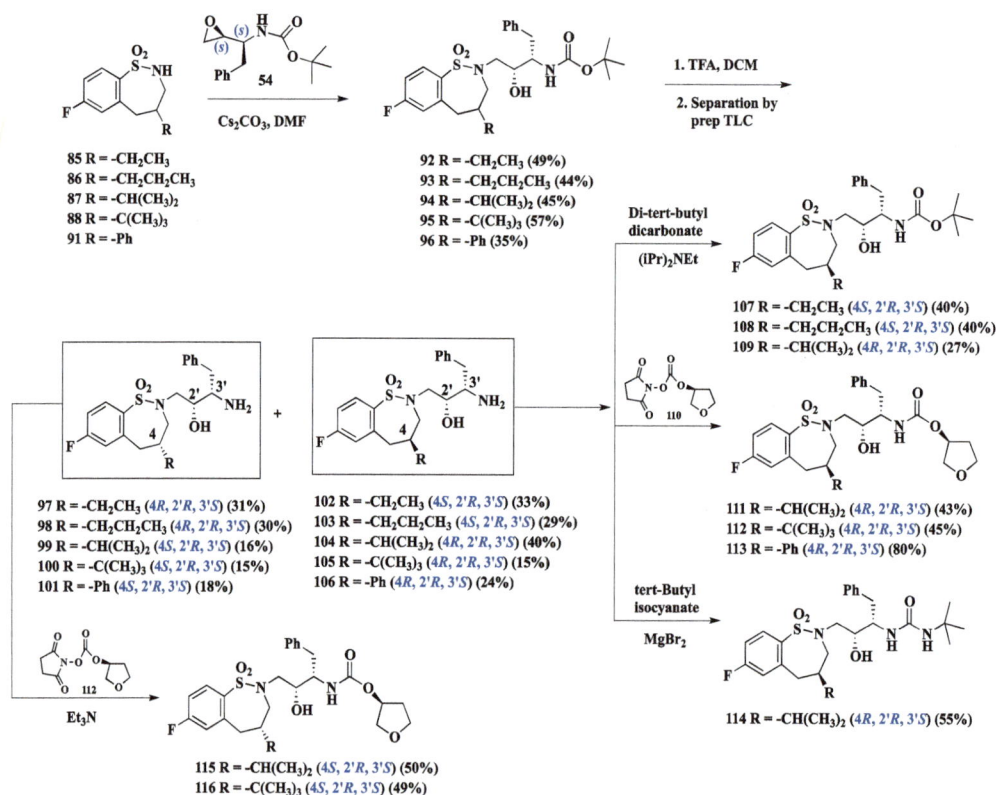

Scheme 14. Synthesis of novel HIV-1 protease inhibitors **107-109, 111-116**.

The X-ray crystal structure of compound **111** bound to the HIV-1 protease is shown in (Fig. 20). It was found that in addition to the binding interactions shown by compound **66**, the tetrahydrofuran group in compound **111** forms a hydrogen bond with Asp 29' and Asp30'. The isopropyl group extends deeper into the hydrophobic pocket of Leu23, Val82, Ile84. It is partially disordered by rotation of the isopropyl group placing the two methyl groups at three positions. The additional interactions are responsible for much improved activity of **111**. The t-butyl group in compound **112** eliminates the disorder of compound **111** and further maximizes the interactions with the hydrophobic pocket, which makes it the most potent analog in this series of compounds. Fig. (**21**) shows overlay of compounds **66, 111** and **114**. Fig. (**22**) shows the overlay of **112** and **116**.

Table 2. Summary of biological activity in HIV-1 protease assay [a]*Replicate of HIV-1 assay at a different time.*

COMPOUND	STRUCTURE	K_i (nM)
Darunavir		<0.02
Amprenavir		0.08 ± 0.02
107		11± 1.1
108		28 ± 6
109		2.8 ± 1.9 3*
111		0.36 ± 0.1 0.43*

(Table 2) cont.....

COMPOUND	STRUCTURE	K_i (nM)
112		0.26 ± 0.05
113		34 ± 5.1
114		6.4 ± 1
115		19 ± 1.6
116		14 ± 0.6

Fig. (20). X-ray crystal structure of compound **111** bound to HIV-1 protease.

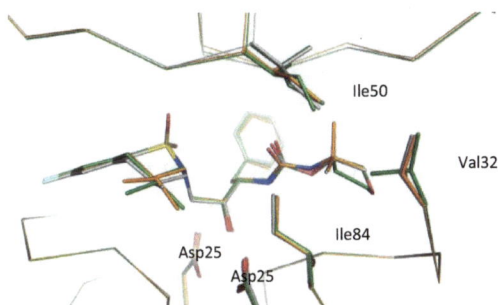

Fig. (21). Overlay of X-ray crystallographic structures of compound **66** (grey), compound **111** (green) and compound **114** (orange).

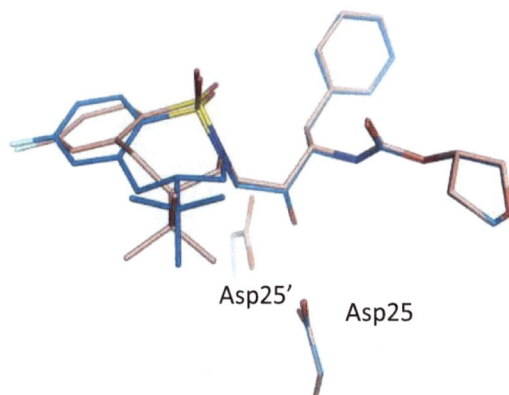

Fig. (22). Overlay of X-ray crystallographic structures of compounds **112** (red) and **116** (blue).

CONCLUSION

In conclusion, we have designed and synthesized a novel class of HIV-1 protease inhibitors bearing a conformationally restricted sulfonamide pharmacophore. The highlights of the synthesis involve an unusual endocyclisation reaction and preparation of analogs with different alkyl and aryl substitution on the cyclic sulfonamide ring. Molecular modeling served as the guide in the initial design of the compounds and the binding interactions of our inhibitors were further confirmed by X-ray crystallographic analysis. We have successfully synthesized several compounds and further optimized the potency to pico molar affinities. The importance of absolute stereochemistry at the three chiral centers for optimum activity was established. Thus compouds with C4-methyl (*S*), C4-ethyl (*S*), C4-propyl (*S*) C4-isopropyl (*R*), C4-t-butyl (*R*) were most potent than their corresponding diastereioisomers, which were inactive/less potent. The compounds with C4-alkyl substitution were significantly more active than the C4-phenyl substitution. The X-ray crystallographic analysis of our compounds **66**, **111** and **112** when bound to the HIV-1 protease enzyme demonstrated that they bind to a similar pocket as in the case of inhibitors such as indinavir/darunavir. These compounds make the key hydrogen bonding interactions to the catalytic aspartic acid residues Asp25 and Asp25' through the 2' hydroxyl group. The sulfonamide and the carbamate carbonyl form hydrogen bonds with a structural water molecule, which in turn hydrogen-bonds with Ile50 and Ile50' of the protease backbone. In addition, the C4 methyl group in compound **66** shows interactions with the hydrophobic pocket containing Leu23, Val82, and Ile84 residues at the active site of the protease enzyme. The C4 isopropyl and t-butyl groups in compounds **111** and **112** further maximize the binding interactions with the catalytic site. Furthermore, the tetrahydrofuran group in compounds **111** and **112** shows hydrogen-bonding interactions with Asp29' and Asp30' of the protease backbone. All the above interactions explain the picomolar activities of our novel inhibitors in the HIV-1 protease assay.

To our greatest surprise we have found that both the C4-iPr (*S*), C4-t-butyl (*S*), **115** and **116** diastereoisomers were active although much less so when compared to the corresponding (*R*) isomers. X-ray studies demonstrated that when bound to the HIV-1 protease they occupy the same pocket as the C4-Me (*S*) diastereoisomer, excepting that in the case of **115** and **116** the seven membered sulfonamide rings assume different conformations. In spite of our best effort we have not been able to get our compounds screened against resistant organisms. It is important that new classes of drugs are discovered as the HIV-1 continues to develop resistance to existing drugs. Currently the HAART regimen involving cocktail of drugs, that inhibit enzymes at various stages in the HIV-1 life cycle, is the most successful treatment for AIDS.

CONSENT FOR PUBLICATION

Not applicable.

CONFLICT OF INTEREST

The authors declare no conflict of interest, financial or otherwise.

ACKNOWLEDGEMENTS

The authors would like to thank Drs Alyssa Antropow, Dipshika Biswas, Alex White, Eric Wang, and Ms Danielle Coroccia, Ms Lacey Samp, who were involved in the synthesis of our work on novel cyclic sulfonamides. Dr. Eunhee Kang, Prof. Yong Zhang for molecular modeling (Stevens), Dr. Li-Kang Zhang for HRMS analysis (Merck). Dr. Steve Caroll, Christine Burlein, Vandana Munshi, John Fay for providing the biological results (Merck). Dr. Corey Strickland, Peter Orth for X-ray crystallography (Merck). We thank Stevens Institute of Technology, Hoboken, NJ, for generous financial support. Some of the material in this chapter has been abstracted from the author's (Sesha Alluri) PhD thesis under the guidance of Prof. A. K. Ganguly.

REFERENCES

[1]   Latest statistics on the status of the AIDs epidemic http://www.unaids.org/en/resources/fact-sheet

[2]   (a). Briz V, Poveda E, Soriano V. HIV entry inhibitors: mechanisms of action and resistance pathways. J Antimicrob Chemother 2006; 57(4): 619-27.
        [http://dx.doi.org/10.1093/jac/dkl027] [PMID: 16464888]
        (b). Lalezari JP, Eron JJ, Carlson M, *et al.* A phase II clinical study of the long-term safety and antiviral activity of enfuvirtide-based antiretroviral therapy. AIDS 2003; 17(5): 691-8.
        [http://dx.doi.org/10.1097/00002030-200303280-00007] [PMID: 12646792]
        (c). Lazzarin A, Clotet B, Cooper D, *et al.* TORO 2 Study Group. Efficacy of enfuvirtide in patients infected with drug-resistant HIV-1 in Europe and Australia. N Engl J Med 2003; 348(22): 2186-95.
        [http://dx.doi.org/10.1056/NEJMoa035211] [PMID: 12773645]

[3]   (a). Kilby JM, Hopkins S, Venetta TM, *et al.* Potent suppression of HIV-1 replication in humans by T-20, a peptide inhibitor of gp41-mediated virus entry. Nat Med 1998; 4(11): 1302-7.
        [http://dx.doi.org/10.1038/3293] [PMID: 9809555]
        (b). Lalezari JP, Luber AD. Enfuvirtide. Drugs Today (Barc) 2004; 40(3): 259-69.
        [http://dx.doi.org/10.1358/dot.2004.40.3.820089] [PMID: 15148534]

[4]   (a). Kuppanna A, Bhaskar MR, Komma R, Datta D. 2011.
        (b). Bray BL. Large-scale manufacture of peptide therapeutics by chemical synthesis. Nat Rev Drug Discov 2003; 2(7): 587-93.
        [http://dx.doi.org/10.1038/nrd1133] [PMID: 12815383]

[5]   Kuritzkes D, Kar S, Kirkpatrick P. Maraviroc. Nat Rev Drug Discov 2008; 7: 15-6.
        [http://dx.doi.org/10.1038/nrd2490]

[6]   (a). Price DA, Gayton S, Selby MD, *et al.* Initial synthesis of UK-427,857 (Maraviroc). Tetrahedron Lett 2005; 46: 5005-7.
        [http://dx.doi.org/10.1016/j.tetlet.2005.05.082]
        (b). Ahman J, Birch M, Haycock-Lewandowski SJ, Long J, Wilder A. Process research and scale-up of a commercialisable route to maraviroc (UK-427,857), a CCR-5 receptor antagonist. Org Process Res Dev 2008; 12: 1104-13.
        [http://dx.doi.org/10.1021/op800062d]

[7]   Mitsuya H, Weinhold KJ, Furman PA, *et al.* 3'-Azido-3'-deoxythymidine (BW A509U): an antiviral agent that inhibits the infectivity and cytopathic effect of human T-lymphotropic virus type III/lymphadenopathy-associated virus *in vitro*. Proc Natl Acad Sci USA 1985; 82(20): 7096-100.
        [http://dx.doi.org/10.1073/pnas.82.20.7096] [PMID: 2413459]

[8]   Czernecki S, Valery JM. An efficient synthesis of 3'-Azido-3'-Deoxythymidine (AZT). Synthesis 1991; 3: 239-40.
        [http://dx.doi.org/10.1055/s-1991-26434]

[9]   Crimmins MT, King BW. An efficient asymmetric approach to carbocyclic nucleosides: Asymmetric synthesis of 1592U89, a potent inhibitor of HIV reverse transcriptase. J Org Chem 1996; 61(13): 4192-3.
        [http://dx.doi.org/10.1021/jo960708p] [PMID: 11667311]

[10]   de Béthune MP. Non-nucleoside reverse transcriptase inhibitors (NNRTIs), their discovery, development, and use in the treatment of HIV-1 infection: a review of the last 20 years (1989-2009). Antiviral Res 2010; 85(1): 75-90.
        [http://dx.doi.org/10.1016/j.antiviral.2009.09.008] [PMID: 19781578]

[11]   Chava S, Ramanjaneyulu G, Indukuri VSK, *et al.* A process for preparation of nevirapine 2012. WO2012168949A2

[12] Joshi S, Maikap GC, Titirmare S, Chaudhari A, Gurjar MK. An improved synthesis of etravirine. Org Process Res Dev 2010; 14(3): 657-60.
[http://dx.doi.org/10.1021/op9003289]

[13] Esposito D, Craigie R. HIV integrase structure and function. Adv Virus Res 1999; 52: 319-33.
[http://dx.doi.org/10.1016/S0065-3527(08)60304-8] [PMID: 10384240]

[14] (a). Patil GD, Kshirsagar SW, Shinde SB, *et al.* Identification, synthesis and strategy for minimization of potential impurities observed in raltegravir potassium drug substance. Org Process Res Dev 2012; 16: 1422-9.
[http://dx.doi.org/10.1021/op300077m]
(b). Pace P, Spieser SAH, Summa V. 4-Hydroxy-5-pyrrolinone-3-carboxamide HIV-1 integrase inhibitors. Bioorg Med Chem Lett 2008; 18(14): 3865-9.
[http://dx.doi.org/10.1016/j.bmcl.2008.06.056] [PMID: 18595690]

[15] Wlodawer A, Vondrasek J. Inhibitors of HIV-1 protease: a major success of structure-assisted drug design. Annu Rev Biophys Biomol Struct 1998; 27: 249-84.
[http://dx.doi.org/10.1146/annurev.biophys.27.1.249] [PMID: 9646869]

[16] (a). Redshaw S, Roberts NA, Thomas GJ. A history of saquinavir, the first human immunodeficiency virus protease inhibitor. Handbook of experimental pharmacologyProteases as targets for therapy 2000; 140: pp. 3-21.;
(b). Lyle TA. 2007.;
(c). Navia MA, Murcko MA. Use of structural information in drug design. Curr Opin Struct Biol. 1992; 2: pp. 202-10.
[http://dx.doi.org/10.1016/0959-440X(92)90147-Y] ;
(d). Raza A, Sham YY, Vince R. Design and synthesis of sulfoximine based inhibitors for HIV-1 protease. Bioorg Med Chem Lett. 2008; 18: pp. (20)5406-10.
[http://dx.doi.org/10.1016/j.bmcl.2008.09.044] [PMID: 18829317] ;
(e). Koh Y, Nakata H, Maeda K, *et al.* Novel bis-tetrahydrofuranylurethane-containing nonpeptidic protease inhibitor (PI) UIC-94017 (TMC114) with potent activity against multi-PI-resistant human immunodeficiency virus *in vitro.*. Antimicrob Agents Chemother. 2003; 47: pp. (10)3123-9.
[http://dx.doi.org/10.1128/AAC.47.10.3123-3129.2003] [PMID: 14506019]

[17] Ghosh AK, Dawson ZL, Mitsuya H. Darunavir, a conceptually new HIV-1 protease inhibitor for the treatment of drug-resistant HIV. Bioorg Med Chem 2007; 15(24): 7576-80.
[http://dx.doi.org/10.1016/j.bmc.2007.09.010] [PMID: 17900913]

[18] Kim EE, Baker CT, Dwyer MD, *et al.* Crystal structure of HIV-1 protease in complex with VX-478, a potent and orally bioavailable inhibitor of the enzyme. J Am Chem Soc 1995; 117(3): 1181-2.
[http://dx.doi.org/10.1021/ja00108a056]

[19] (a). Vellanki SRP, Sahu A, Phadhuri NK, Kilaru R. Crystalline darunavir 2013. WO2013114382A1
(b). Moore GL, Stringham RW, Teager DS, Yue TY. Practical synthesis of the bicyclic darunavir side chain: (3R, 3aS, 6aR)-Hexahydrofuro[2,3-b]furan-3-ol from monopotassium isocitrate. Org Process Res Dev 2017; 21(1): 98-106.
[http://dx.doi.org/10.1021/acs.oprd.6b00377] [PMID: 28539755]

[20] Ghosh AK, Chapsal BD, Baldridge A, *et al.* Design and synthesis of potent HIV-1 protease inhibitors incorporating hexahydrofuropyranol-derived high affinity $P_{(2)}$ ligands: structure-activity studies and biological evaluation. J Med Chem 2011; 54(2): 622-34.
[http://dx.doi.org/10.1021/jm1012787] [PMID: 21194227]

[21] (a). Ganguly AK, Alluri SS, Caroccia D, *et al.* Design, synthesis, and X-ray crystallographic analysis of a novel class of HIV-1 protease inhibitors. J Med Chem 2011; 54(20): 7176-83.
[http://dx.doi.org/10.1021/jm200778q] [PMID: 21916489]
(b). Ganguly AK, Alluri SS, Wang C-H, *et al.* Structural optimization of cyclic sulfonamide based novel HIV-1 protease inhibitors to picomolar affinities guided by X-ray crystallographic analysis. Tetrahedron 2014; 70: 2894-904.

[http://dx.doi.org/10.1016/j.tet.2014.03.038]

[22]   Ghosh AK, Sean Fyvie W, Brindisi M, *et al.* Design, synthesis, X-ray studies, and biological evaluation of novel macrocyclic HIV-1 protease inhibitors involving the P1′-P2′ ligands. Bioorg Med Chem Lett 2017; 27(21): 4925-31.
       [http://dx.doi.org/10.1016/j.bmcl.2017.09.003] [PMID: 28958624]

[23]   Biswas D, Samp L, Ganguly AK. Synthesis of conformationally restricted sulfonamides *via* radical cyclisation. Tetrahedron Lett 2010; 51: 2681-4.
       [http://dx.doi.org/10.1016/j.tetlet.2010.03.089]

[24]   Hohlfeld K, Tomassi C, Wegner JK, Kesteleyn B, Linclau B. Disubstituted bis-THF moieties as new P2 ligands in nonpeptidal HIV-1 protease inhibitors. ACS Med Chem Lett 2011; 2(6): 461-5.
       [http://dx.doi.org/10.1021/ml2000356] [PMID: 24900331]

CHAPTER 2

Potential Magnetic Nanotherapeutics for Management of neuroAIDS

Vidya Sagar*, Arti Vashist and Madhavan Nair*

Center for Personalized Nanomedicine/Institute of Neuroimmune Pharmacology, Department of Immunology, Herbert Wertheim College of Medicine, Florida International University, Miami, Florida - 33199, USA

Abstract: The human immunodeficiency virus (HIV) infection into the brain induces neurotoxicity and neuropathology which are collectively termed as the neuroAIDS. Brain delivery of therapeutic molecules continues to be the greatest challenge, primarily because of the tightly-junctioned blood-brain barrier (BBB). Several nano-vehicles are under intensive examination for delivering drugs across the BBB. Magnetic nanoparticles (MNPs) possess advantages over their counterparts because of their potential utilization for non-invasive brain targeting using external magnetic force. MNPs can be physicochemically modulated for engineering smart drug delivery carrier as well. Nonetheless, rigorous research is required to fix associated shortcomings of MNPs before their real-time application.

Keywords: Blood-Brain Barrier, HIV, Magnetic Nanocarriers, NeuroAIDS, Neuropathogenesis, Synaptic plasticity.

MECHANISMS OF NEUROAIDS

Neuroinvasion by human immunodeficiency virus (HIV) is initiated early during infection which leads to gradual appearance and progression of neurologic conditions of different intensities. The collective neurological condition of HIV patients is termed as "neuroAIDS". Nonetheless, HIV is not solely responsible for this condition; rather opportunistic bacterial, fungal, and/or viral infections and toxic effects of anti-HIV drugs also contribute to a significant level in aggravating neuroAIDS conditions [1, 2]. The phenotypic appearance of neuroAIDS is reflected as downgraded learning and information processing ability which can be correlated with the deterioration of associated brain regions and spinal cord of HIV patients. While the phenotypic appearance of only 50% patients

* Corresponding authors Vidya Sagar and Madhavan Nair: Center for Personalized Nanomedicine/Institute of Neuroimmune Pharmacology, Department of Immunology, Herbert Wertheim College of Medicine, Florida International University, Miami, Florida - 33199, USA; Tel/Fax: +1-305-348-1491; E-mails: vsaga001@fiu.edu; nairm@fiu.edu

Atta-ur-Rahman (Ed.)

demonstrates neurological symptoms of some kind; a more serious scenario is noticeable upon autopsies where ~80% of AIDS patients show mild to severe neurological deformities [3, 4]. Neurological complications of neuroAIDS conditions range from dementia, peripheral neuropathies, chronic meningitis, and neurosyphilis to CNS lymphomas, progressive multifocal leukoencephalopathy, and vacuolar myelopathy. Several other neurological deformities of known and unknown origin are also seen in HIV patients [1, 5 - 8]. The enigma of neuroAIDS continues from the initial phase to late phase of HIV infection and is filled with multifaceted symptoms and pathologies. It is hard to find a precise diagnosis for neuroAIDS and associated complexities in HIV patients and it will continue till the discovery of specific diagnosis tools and/or protocols. In initial years, HIV presence in the brain during early and/or late infection was determined based on detection of particles, proteins, and genetic components of HIV in the CNS and intrathecal production of anti-HIV antibodies as well [9, 10]. Confirmation of the early presence of HIV in the brain by these studies opened the way for examining mechanisms of HIV entry into the brain. It is putatively believed that entry of HIV into the brain is mediated by transendothelial migration of infected mononuclear phagocytes, especially monocytes and blood-borne macrophages. Transmigration of these cells across the blood-brain barrier (BBB) lies in their intrinsic ability to migrate towards specific cytokines/chemokines-stimulation (*e.g.* monocyte chemotactic protein-1) [11, 12]. Initial migration of HIV-infected cells to the brain and subsequent infection triggers the release of those factors which weaken the BBB integrity (*e.g.* matrix metalloproteinase) [13, 14]. This induces an influx of inflammation responsive leukocytes into the brain. The influxed cell populations include both infected and non-infected leukocytes at an increased rate, and consequently, more HIV-infected cells are accumulated in the brain resulting in the disease intensification and spread of HIV infection in other brain cell types as well [7, 15, 16]. While susceptibility of astrocytes and microglia to HIV infection has been well established, the ability of HIV to invade nerve cells continues to be an area of debate. A subpopulation of almost all kind of HIV-infected cells including brain cells acquires latency in such a way that HIV in these cell subpopulation experiences no deleterious effect of cellular immune response and antiretroviral drugs. Latent cells exert zero and/or minimum transcription of host-integrated HIV genome and thus no or little virus is produced in comparison to active cells. Latent HIV infection can persist for years resulting in chronic pathological implications [17]. Also, it can continuously rebind viremia in patients upon reactivation. Latent cells can be reactivated by specific endogenous or exogenous latency-breaking stimulus [10]. Thus, both latent and active HIV infection contributes toward the neuroAIDS condition.

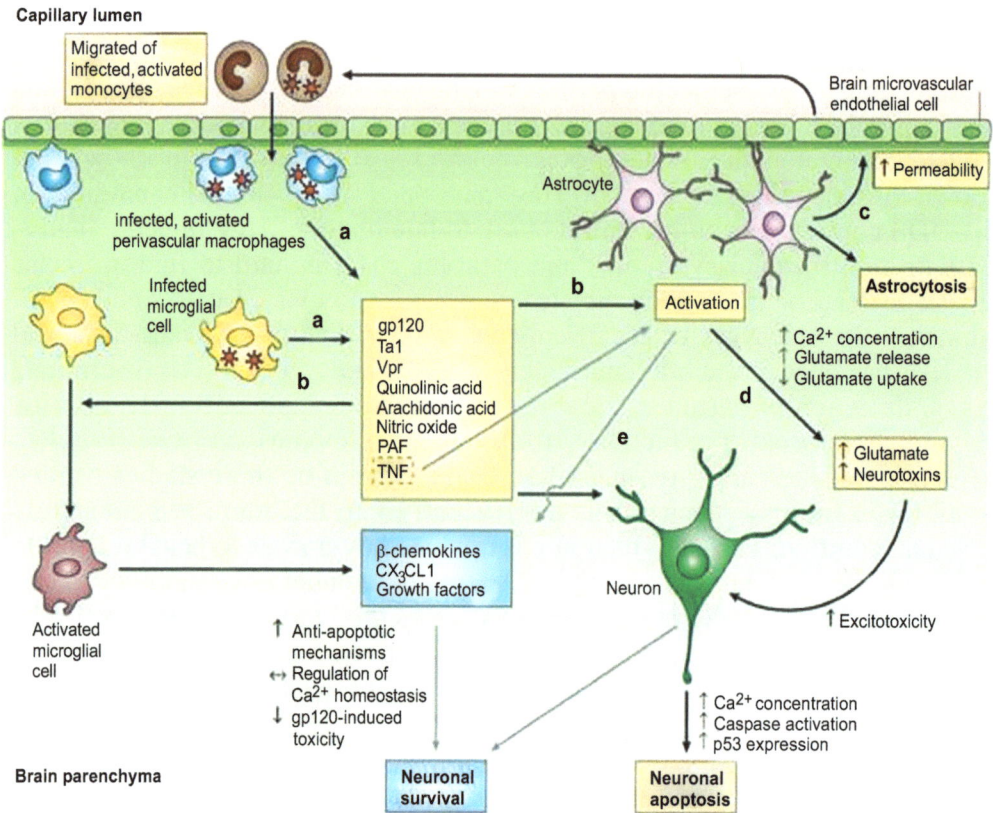

Fig. (1). Mechanisms of neuroAIDS and potential Neuroprotection **a)** neuroinvasion by HIV-infected perivascular macrophages and microglia and subsequent production of HIV viremia and viral proteins cause deleterious effects on the central nervous system. Neurotoxic proteins of HIV (gp120, Tat, Vpr, Nef, *etc.*) exert adverse effects on different brain cells. Production of inflammatory factors such as cytokines, quinolinic and arachidonic acid, platelet-activating factor, nitric oxide, *etc.* further aggravate the neurotoxic effects. **b)** Neuropathogenesis process also includes activation and/or proliferation of macrophages, microglia, and astrocytes. **c)** These activation and proliferation intensify the production of inflammatory factors and permeability of BBB is compromised. Disturbance of BBB integrity promotes migration of infected and non-infected monocytes into the brain. Thus infected macrophages are accumulated in higher concentration. **d)** The whole process eventually causes neuronal apoptosis and the mechanism involves an increase in the intracellular Ca^{2+}, p53 expression, glutamate release, neurotoxin production, excitotoxicity, and caspase activation. **e)** Intrinsically brain also activates survival mechanism during viral insults, nonetheless, neurotoxic effect dominates over the survival mechanisms in most cases. The neuroprotective mechanisms (in gray arrow) include the production of tumor necrosis factor and subsequent release of beta-chemokines, CX3C-chemokine ligand 1 (CX3CL1), and growth factors. These factors are known to positively regulate the Ca^{2+} homeostasis in neurons and promote anti-apoptotic signaling pathways and reduce excitotoxicity. (Reprinted with permission from {González-Scarano F, Martín-García J. The neuropathogenesis of AIDS. Nat. Rev. Immunol. 2005;5:69–81}, Copyright {2005} Nature Publishing Group).

At the molecular level neuroAIDS condition is driven by the cumulative deleterious effect of HIV virion and its neurotoxic proteins on different brain cells (Fig. **1**). Every cell types behave differently during HIV infection and, in turn, their molecular cascades are unique. Entry of HIV-infected cells into the brain and their subsequent differentiation, especially of HIV-infected monocytes into macrophages, cause activation of astrocytes and microglia leading to neuroinflammation. Subsequently neuron-damaging, pro-inflammatory molecules such as reactive oxygen species, nitric oxide, TNF-α, IL-1β, *etc.* are released which exacerbate the existing pathogenesis [7, 18]. The presence of HIV gp120 protein further induces the release of these factors in macrophages and microglia and activates chemokine receptors in neurons which cause elevation of intracellular Ca^{2+} concentration and subsequently apoptosis is initiated. The gp120 protein also downregulates glutamate uptake and induces nitric oxide synthase production in astrocytes leading to excitotoxicity and cell death. The role of gp120 in apoptosis of brain microvascular endothelial cells (BMVECs) (BBB disintegration) and inhibition of migration and proliferation of neural progenitor cells (NPCs) have been outlined as well. Similar to gp120, other neurotoxic proteins of HIV, tat, vpr, and nef has a significant role in modulating the molecular landscape and stimulates hostile conditions for different brain cells (Fig. **1**) [2, 7, 18]. In recent years we have examined the synaptodendritic injury during HIV infection by measuring neuronal spine density, dendritic diameter, total spine, and dendritic area. Morphology of neuronal cells is significantly compromised during HIV infections and this is well-correlated with altered expression of genes responsible for the synaptic plasticity regulations [19 - 21]. In the same line, atrophy of gray and white matter is observed in the brain of HIV patients [22]. Thus, one can say that while antiretrovirals delivery into the brain may help in HIV progression, a practical therapeutic regimen for neuroAIDS should also include neuroprotection or neuron-resuscitating agents and a drug that can break the latency phenomenon as well.

CHALLENGES OF BLOOD-BRAIN BARRIER (BBB) FOR NEUROAIDS TREATMENTS

Similar to other brain disorders, two major challenges of neuroAIDS treatments are the presence of BBB and lack of appropriate experimental BBB model. The uniqueness of BBB resides in the anatomical organization of tightly-junctioned BMVECs and choroid epithelial cells which are extended in a fenestrationless manner all along the capillary linings of cerebral microvasculature. The complex of BBB also includes persistent and intimate contact of BMVECs to pericytes and perivascular astrocytes. The structural integrity of BBB complex is maintained by several factors where three tight junction transmembrane integral proteins, namely, occludin, claudin, and junction adhesion molecules play a major role.

Many cytoplasmic accessory proteins, such as cingulin, zonula occludens, 7H6 antigen, *etc.* are equally important. The tightness of transendothelial junction is equivalent to an electrical resistance of 1500-2000 $\Omega c/m^2$ which is 50-100 times higher than that of peripheral blood vessels. The structural organization allows BBB a unique functional ability as an interface to separate the brain parenchyma from the bloodstream [15, 23, 24]. By doing so, BBB allows entry of only selected molecules necessary to maintain the ideal functional efficiency of the brain and therefore safeguards the brain from the peripheral insult. Molecules which are allowed to enter into cerebral space are certain amino acids, monocarboxylic acids, sugars, purine bases, amines, hydrophilic molecules such as O_2 and CO_2, certain neurotransmitters and small lipophilic xenobiotics or endogenous molecules of ≤ 600Da. These molecules, in a case-specific manner, can diffuse transcellularly across the BBB or can be actively transported *via* mechanisms such as carrier-mediated transport, receptors-mediated or absorptive-mediated endocytosis, fluid-phase endocytosis, *etc.* Also, the presence of substrate specific transporters, for example, monocarboxylate transport system, insulin receptor, ceruloplasmin receptor, glucose transporter-1, transferrin receptor, *etc.* allow transportation of their substrate in cerebral space [25 - 27]. However, all these modes of transendothelial transportation and selective permeability of molecules provide very little or no benefit in managing brain diseases because drugs molecules are usually larger in size than the permissible limit and/or have adverse chemical properties than those allowed for transmigrating across BBB. In fact, more than 98% of drug molecules cannot cross the BBB [28]. BBB possess a large spectrum of influx–efflux pumps that can actively transport molecules in or out of the brain. Most antiretroviral (ARV) drugs are either substrate of efflux transporters or inhibitor of influx transporters and therefore their CNS entry is either inaccessible or blocked. Also, BMVECs of BBB (cerebral microvessels) possess a unique set of enzymatic activities (*e.g.* γ-glutamyl transpeptidase, aromatic acid decarboxylase, alkaline phosphatase, *etc.*) for metabolization of undesirable neuroactive substances recruited through peripheral circulation. These enzymes serve as an enzymatic barrier and their luminal or abluminal expression significantly modulates the dynamics and kinetics of xenobiotics in the brain [25, 27, 29 - 31]. The structural and functional sophistication of the BBB are primarily evolved for maintaining brain homeostasis and in turn level of drugs or other exogenous molecules in cerebral space remain either at zero level or are pharmacologically insignificant.

Examining the role/condition of BBB in driving CNS disorders including neuroAIDS in the real-time situation is not possible because of the non-existence of technology that can open brain without deleterious effect. Most study in neuroAIDS utilizes brain samples from dead patients to understand the real-time pathologies. While post-mortem brain study is very useful, it only provides a snapshot of end-stage pathology and details of mechanistic progression of disease from its inception remain unknown [32]. For this purpose, uses of existing *in vitro* or *in vivo* models for therapeutical study are prevalent. However, these models have many demerits which prevent them to mimic real-time functional BBB in human. Especially, the BBB dynamics to different kind of physiological disturbances throughout disease progression is hard to mimic [10, 33]. One of the most popular approaches utilizes *in vitro* BBB model where endothelial cells are co-cultured with astrocytes and pericytes. The onset of BBB formation is driven by the presence of other surrounding cell and tissue microenvironment as well which are lacking in this model. For example, contact of endothelial cells with neural stem cells and physical and mechanical stimuli generated by various kinds of cell-to-cell contacts are major modulators of endothelial cells during BBB formation [10, 33, 34]. Simplified understanding obtained through this model must be assessed in *in vivo* systems. In this context, the major hurdle is the lack of suitable humanized rodent model for neuroAIDS. Existing rodent models for neuroAIDS possess several caveats and are questionable to a greater extent [35]. Currently, macaque model system is believed to be the more pertinent animal models for neuroAIDS study. Nonetheless, different characteristics of simian virus strain in compare to human strain and different susceptibility and pharmacokinetics of macaque than human are few factors that limit the use of this model from developing effective therapeutics for neuroAIDS [10, 32, 36]. Similar to several microbial pathogeneses where humanized rodent models have led to successful therapeutics, efforts are being taken toward humanization of the mouse for neuroAIDS within the boundary of biological and economical sophistication so that they can have reach across maximum laboratories for intensive research.

ADVANTAGES OF NANOTHERAPEUTICS FOR MANAGEMENT OF NEUROAIDS

In the last two decades, several approaches have been strategized and trialed to send an adequate amount of antiretrovirals across the BBB. For example, ATP-binding cassette (ABC) transporters blocking approach uses inhibitors against specific efflux receptors at BBB in order to make higher brain delivery of those ARV drugs which are a substrate of these efflux receptors. The presence of ABC transporters across different body organs or tissues reduces the CNS-specificity of this approach and higher ARV transportation to different tissue can cause toxicity as well [31, 37 - 39]. Some ARV prodrugs have been identified to gain access to perivascular and meningeal macrophages *via* blood-cerebrospinal fluid barrier of the choroid plexus. Nonetheless, prodrugs are only effective if they are metabolized to its effective form in the body [10, 40 - 42]. Further, focused ultrasound and microbubble approach have been applied toward the transient opening of BBB [43, 44]. Similarly, hyperosmotic solutions [45] and intra-arterial delivery of vasoactive agents [46 - 48] have been examined for disrupting the BBB permeability. However, BBB opening in these cases cannot be manually controlled and therefore the passage of undesirable molecules into the brain can result in severe neuro-damaging insults. Recently, nanoscale technology-based drug delivery approaches have emerged as attractive options to be emulated for the development of novel nanoformulations with the ability to treat neurodisorders. Several types of nanoformulations have been developed for treating neuroAIDS (Fig. **2**).

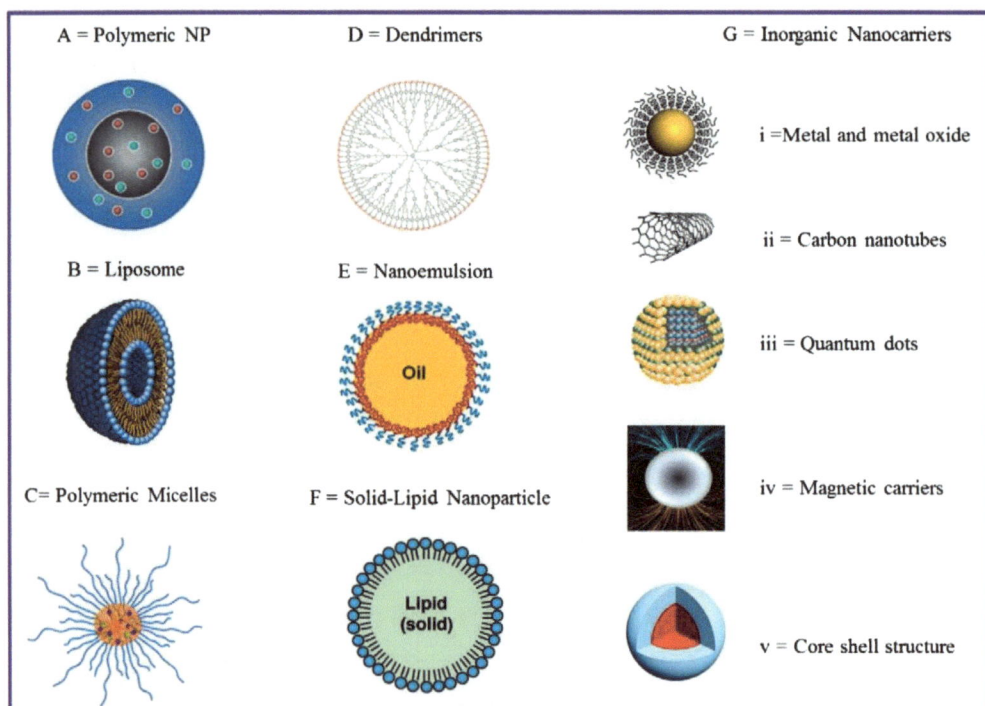

Fig. (2). Depiction of various nanocarrier systems for potential brain targeting [2].
(Reprinted with permission from {Nair M, Jayant RD, Kaushik A, *et al.* Getting into the brain: Potential of nanotechnology in the management of NeuroAIDS. Adv. Drug Deliv. Rev. 2016;103:202–217.}, Copyright {2016} Elsevier B.V.).

Materials at their nanometer size range acquire unique physicochemical properties. Especially, their higher specific surface area makes them ideal for the drug delivery carrier. Nonetheless, several other properties of nanomaterials are combinedly utilized for drug delivery. Higher specific surface area adds to their drug loading ability which, in turn, improves the drug dissolution rate and release kinetics such that an initial burst release is followed by a constant slow release. Similarly, material's crystallinity modulates their dissolution characteristics where amorphous region degrades faster than the crystalline region. Accordingly, drug's release kinetics from nanocarriers follows dissolution pattern with faster and slower release one after other. Also, nanocarrier's surface charge plays a significant role in drug loading and release kinetics. The intrinsic surface charge of nanocarriers or charge developed by surface coatings influences the nanocarriers-drug association such that hydrophobicity prolongs drug release. Hydrophobicity also prolongs the blood circulation time. Hydrophilic surface property improves nanocarrier's ability to bind with poorly soluble drugs. Maintaining size of ≤100 nm is equally significant aspects of nanocarriers because particles within this size can escape the reticuloendothelial (RES) circulation and therefore their first-pass hepatic metabolism can be minimized resulting in increased bioavailability. Nanocarriers also gain the ability to freely flow into the capillaries and therefore can reach to every nook and corner of the body with increased circulation time. Nanosized particles also show higher intracellular uptake which makes them transmigrate across different physiological barriers (*e.g.* stomach epithelial barrier). Surface charge distribution further adds to the cellular uptake of nanocarriers. While the positive charge of nanocarriers can easily interact with the natural negative charge of the cell membrane, hydrophilic nanocarriers can circumvent opsonization. Functionally, the concept of nano-drug is strategized for target-specific, safe, and controllable drug-delivery. Nano-carriers can be modulated for both passive and active targeting. Application of nanocarriers for active targeting is prevalent where drug-loaded nanocarriers are tethered with the target-specific moieties. Nanocarriers with active targeting ability can provide better efficacy and lesser side effects. The passive targeting utilizes two important characteristics of nanocarriers, reduced first-pass hepatic metabolism and increased blood circulation time. A famous example of nanocarrier-mediated passive targeting is enhanced permeability and retention effect in targeting tumors of the enterohepatic circuit. HIV infections of lymph nodes can also be targeted using the passive targeting [10,49 - 51]].

Overall, an ideal nanocarrier system must have a certain sets of characteristics such as, for example, a) should be soluble, non-toxic and biocompatible; b) should not block the blood vessels, achieve long circulation time, and have longer bioavailability as well; c) should provide protection to bound drugs from the peripheral enzymatic and hydrolytic degradation; and d) should provide ability to control the delivery and release of drugs to achieve timely onset of therapeutic action at the target [2].

MAGNETIC NANOTHERAPEUTICS FOR MANAGEMENT OF NEUROAIDS

Complying with the notion of nanocarriers system, several drug delivery approaches have been applied towards better ARV distribution to the brain. Both passive and active targeting ability of nanocarriers have been opined. The hypothesis of passive targeting recommends for the higher accumulation of drug at endothelium of BBB to create local gradient difference for passive transendothelial diffusion of drugs [31]. In some cases, nonreceptor-mediated endocytosis (*e.g.* macropinocytosis) may increase cellular drug trafficking. Active drug targeting utilizes receptor-mediated endocytosis by tethering receptor-specific ligand or uses efflux transporters inhibitors or blocking agent to the nanocarrier's surface [10]. These hypotheses made the basis for engineering some exciting nano-vehicles with wider theranostics applications and currently many are under investigations with updated features. Nonetheless, existing nano-vehicles (*e.g.* liposomes, dendrimers, polymers, micelles, solid-lipid particles, *etc.*) possess several limitations with respect to transendothelial targeting (Table 1). One major issue is their susceptibility to extensive first pass metabolism or uptake by RES cells. These nanocarriers stay in peripheral circulation for longer time and majority of them are lost in different organs before reaching to brain vasculature. Studies have shown that most of these carriers are deposited either in liver, lungs or other lymphoid organs [50]. It should be noted that ARVs have short elimination half-life and therefore their prolonged stay in the periphery can remarkably reduce the bioavailability and pharmacokinetics [31, 10, 52]. Hence, effective drug targeting to the brain requires rapid and organized transport of carriers to the target before they get engulfed by RES.

Table 1. A comparison of different nanocarrier system for brain targeting during HIV infection: Most of these targeting strategies are in preclinical laboratory stages and therefore intensive research involving numerous trials and errors is required for the extension of technologies to the next level of experimentation [10].
(Reprinted with permission from {Sagar V, Pilakka-Kanthikeel S, Pottathil R, *et al.* Towards nanomedicines for neuroAIDS. Rev. Med. Virol. 2014;24:103–124}, Copyright {2014} the John Wiley and Sons, Ltd.).

Nanoparticle types	BBB Transmigration Potential	Limitations	Suggested Improvements
Polymers	• Increased transmigration of ARV drugs across *in vitro* BBB and mouse model.	• Not ideal for the delivery of polar/ionic compounds. • Transient inflammation may occur.	• Nanocarrier potential of natural polymers should be intensively explored.
Dendrimers	• Increased transmigration of antiviral siRNA across *in vitro* BBB.	• Complex synthesis process. • Inconsistent and premature drug release. • Polycationic moieties cause cytotoxicity.	• More *in vitro* and *in vivo* transmigration assays are essentially required. • Toxicity of different neuronal cells must be well defined.

(Table 1) contd.....

Nanoparticle types	BBB Transmigration Potential	Limitations	Suggested Improvements
Micelle	• Increased transmigration and efficacy of ARV drugs across *in vitro* BBB and mouse model.	• Particles are comparatively unstable which results in premature drug release.	• Brain-specific ligand tethering may improve the active targeting.
Liposomes	• Could be developed as "Trojan nanocarrier" residing in the monocytes/macrophages which naturally transmigrate across BBB. • Increased transmigration of ARV drugs across *in vitro* BBB and rat model.	• Possess low drug entrapment ability. • Inefficient loading of water-soluble drugs. • Instability and leakiness of loaded drugs during storage.	• Surface charge modifications such as PEGlyation can improve stability • Brain tissue-specific antibodies /ligands conjugation could enhance active targeting.
Solid-lipid	• Increased transmigration of ARV drugs across *in vitro* BBB model.	• Limited *in vivo* study to show its lab-to-land transferability.	• More *in vitro* and *in vivo* transmigration study required to authenticate its applicability.
Magnetic	• Could by hybridize with liposomes as "Magneto-liposomes" which can behave as "Trojan magneto-liposomes" residing in monocyte/macrophage. • Externally magnetic force mediated movement helps in the escape of nanocarriers' uptake from the reticuloendothelial system and accelerates active targeting. • Increased transmigration of ARV drugs across *in vitro* BBB model.	• Though many *in vivo* study showed site-specific targeting and lab-to-land transferability for non-HIV drugs, the same for ARV drugs are very limited.	• More *in vivo* study based on mouse, rat, or monkey models must be performed.
Cell-based	• ARV drugs loaded on nanocarriers and their packaging in macrophage (which can cross BBB paracellularly) show increased transmigration and antiretroviral efficacy across *in vitro* BBB and mice model.	• Drug release mechanism from the cellular carrier at the delivered site is an area which is less understood. • Possible cytotoxicity at targeted area *via* production of reactive oxygen species by inflammatory-response cells such as monocytes, macrophages *etc*.	• Transmigration ability of many other inflammatory-response cells such as dendritic cells, neuronal stem cells, *etc.* may lead to finding a better cellular carrier. • Tethering of cellular specific receptors to nanocarriers may mimic the cellular carrier and in turn, cell-based cytotoxicity could be minimized.

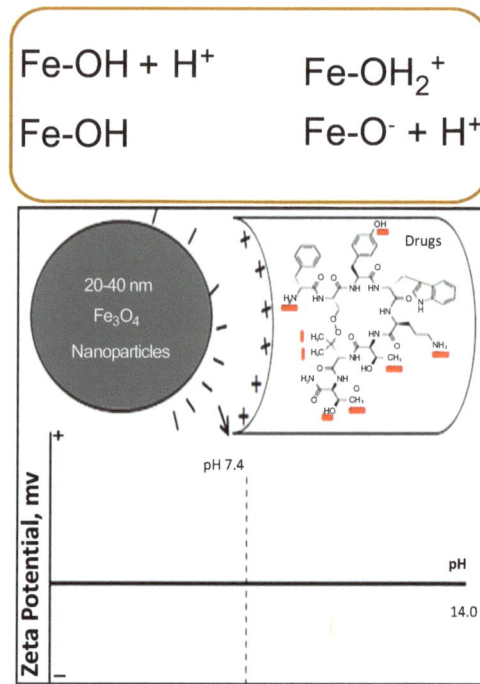

Fig. (3). Depiction of drugs interaction with MNPs [59]: Protonation and deprotonation on MNPs surface allow direct binding of biomolecules/molecules. MNPs (Fe_3O_4) in aqueous solutions perform amphoterism due to adsorption of amphoteric "-OH" group and develop positive or negative charges at the magnetite-water interface in pH- dependent manner. MNPs develop significant negative charge at pH 7.4 and therefore positively charged molecules can interact *via* ionic bonding. Charges on the MNPs surface can be modulated by surfactant coatings as per the necessity.
Reprinted with permission from {Sagar V, Pilakka-Kanthikeel S, Atluri VSR, *et al.* Therapeutical neurotargeting *via* magnetic nanocarrier: Implications to opiate-induced neuropathogenesis and NeuroAIDS. J. Biomed. Nanotechnol. 2015;11:1722–1733.}, Copyright {2000-2017} American Scientific Publishers).

Recently magnetic nanoparticles (MNPs) have gained significant attention and have shown great promise in imaging and drug targeting. In most cases, magnetite (Fe_3O_4) and maghemite (Υ-Fe_2O_3) have been investigated for target-specific drug delivery. The superparamagnetism of MNPs provides them unique ability to be utilized for simultaneous actuation and imaging purpose. Movement of MNPs can be directed toward desired targets using external "remote" magnetic field [52] and magnetic moment induced intrinsic proton signal in the periphery of MNPs can be utilized for contrast agent in magnetic resonance imaging [53]. Thus, both movement and tissue distribution of MNPs and its associated molecules can be monitored and quantitated. This can help in optimizing site-specific drug dosing. Many of MNP's other characteristics are equally indispensable for a drug delivery carrier. Easiness in laboratory synthesis of MNPs allows production of monodispersed particles with flexible size range as per requirement. Here again, higher surface to volume ratio of particles enhances target affinity which helps them to manipulate even at subcellular levels [10]. MNPs (especially Fe_3O_4) displays amphoterism in aqueous solutions and therefore positive or negative charge on their surface can be developed in a pH-dependent manner [54] (Fig. **3**). This provides flexibility to modulate surface charge for direct or indirect binding of a wide range of molecules. MNPs can also be encapsulated into liposomes which have been termed as "magnetoliposomes" (Fig. **4B**) [55, 56].

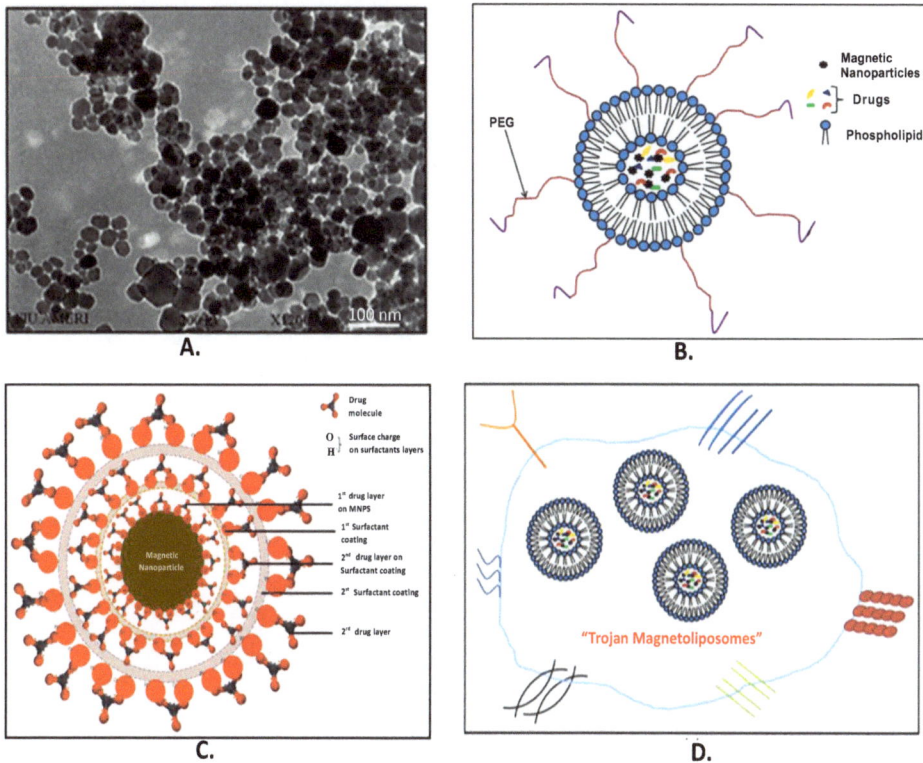

Fig. (4). Different forms of MNPs nanocarriers for delivery of ARVs across BBB: (**A**) TEM imaging of MNPs [10]. (**B**) Magnetoliposomes - MNPs bound ARV drugs are encapsulated in liposomes. The carrier surface is tethered with PEG which provides stability and enhances circulation time [10]. (**C**) Magnetic layer-by-layer assembly- MNPs are used as a solid platform to build alternate layers of polymers and drugs [18, 60]. (**D**) Magnetized cell-mediated drug delivery: Magnetoliposomes are packaged into monocytes/macrophages [10]. These magnetized cells can naturally travel to the zone of inflammation or magnetic field can also direct them to the targeted area.
(Fig A-B & D: Reprinted with permission from {Sagar V, Pilakka-Kanthikeel S, Pottathil R, *et al.* Towards nanomedicines for neuroAIDS. Rev. Med. Virol. 2014;24:103–124}, Copyright {2014} The John Wiley and Sons, Ltd.; Fig C: BioMed Central allow re-use of content in any way, subject only to proper attribution.)

Magnetoliposomes have several advantages, such as, for example, per unit loading efficiency of nanocarrier is enhanced because additional drugs can be loaded on phospholipids and liposomal core as well, encapsulated drugs can be protected from the enzymatic and hydrolytic degradation in peripheral circulation which results in increased drug bioavailability, *etc* [10, 56, 57]. Similar to MNPs, movement of magnetoliposomes can be manipulated by external magnetic force. Toxicity must be a vital consideration during nanoparticles application. In this context, MNPs are biodegradable and reflects non-significant safety concern within the permissible dose limit [58]. All these features of MNPs can mold it to be used for brain-targeted drug delivery where therapeutic molecules of all kind (*e.g.* proteins, enzymes, drugs, siRNAs, *etc.*) can be immobilized on the carriers.

Application of MNPs for neuroAIDS targeting are at early pre-clinical stages and have shown significant potential for their extension to the next level of experimentation. Our team has extensively studied MNPs for sending ARVs across BBB. In a very first attempt, a magnetic nanoformulation of 3′-azido-3′ - deoxythymidine-5′ -triphosphate (AZTTP) was encapsulated in liposomes for *in vitro* BBB transmigration assay. The magneto-liposomal nanoformulations showed nearly 3 fold higher transendothelial migrations and anti-HIV potency of AZTTP was intact for at least 14 days of experimental period [56]. Dextran sulfate based layer-by-layer magnetic nanoformulations (Fig. **4C**) of Tenofovir was developed to achieve sustained release of drugs for ≥ 5 days. This formulation showed 2.8 times higher drug loading ability and its *in vitro* transendothelial migration increased by nearly 38%. The efficacy of this layer-b--layer nanoformulation remained intact for 5 days where ~ 33% reduction in HIV replication was noticed [60]. In another study amphiphilic polymer [poly (isobutylene-alt-1-tetradecene-maleic anhydride] was coated on MNPs surface to increase the translocation of nanoformulation across BBB. This mouse-based study showed successful delivery of ARV, Enfuvirtide in the brain [61]. Several brain targeting fraction of HIV or non-HIV peptides have been used for surface coating on magnetic nanocarriers. Tethering of Tat peptide fraction on the surface of magneto-liposomal nanoformulations can be effective in brain drug delivery [62]. Similarly, a fraction of the Nef peptide with myristoylation site (known to prevent the release of deleterious Nef-containing exosome from brain cells) was nanoformulated with the MNPs. The nanoformulations showed efficacy in preventing BBB integrity during HIV infection and therefore it could potentially reduce the HIV-associated neuropathogenesis [63]. Notably, all these nanoformulations were nontoxic and did not alter the BBB integrity. Thus, HIV targeted magnetic nanoformulations showed promise in preventing HIV pathogenesis in brain cells.

As stated earlier, HIV causes significant injury to neurons and therefore effective therapeutics for neuroAIDS must be supplemented with the neuroprotective agents. A magnetic nanoformulation of the neuroprotective agent (TMP-1) showed an increase in spinal density with reduced HIV replication. In this case, transmigration of nanoformulation across *in vitro* BBB was increased by ~ 40% [64]. In a unique study, magnetic nanoformulations of brain-derived neurotropic factor (BDNF) were developed to protect the neuronal damage in morphine-treated cells during HIV infection [65].

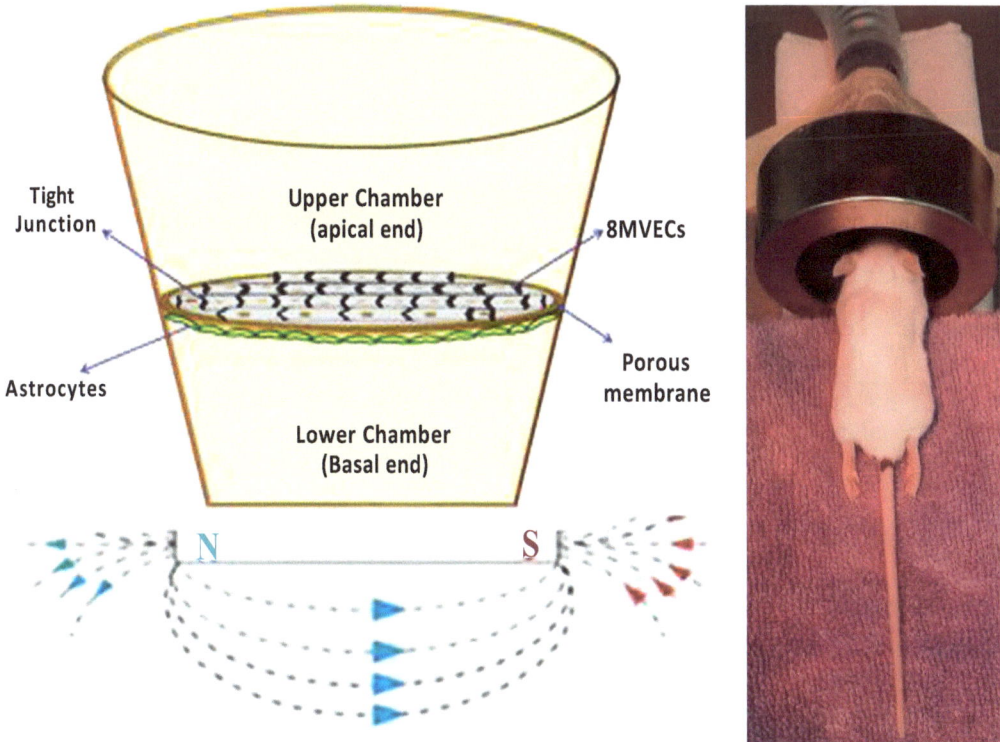

Fig. (5). MNPs transmigration across BBB [18]: **A)** Most commonly used *in vitro* BBB model is based on co-culture of astrocytes and endothelial cells in a bi-compartmentalized transwell plate. The porous membrane of the transwell is cultured with the tightly-junctioned endothelial cells on its top and underside of the membrane is cultured with astrocytes. This mimicked from of BBB is placed on top of the magnetic field which influence migration of MNPs from the upper chamber to lower chamber. **(B)** In a rodent model, brain targeting using MNPs involves intravenous injection of MNPs to anesthetized animal followed by exposure of desired magnetic field for a specific time by positioning head between the poles of the magnetic coil. (BioMed Central allows re-use of content in any way, subject only to proper attribution).

It should be noted that spread of HIV infection and progression of neuroAIDS is significantly influenced by recreation drug abuse. Nearly 10% of HIV patients suffer from the addiction of one or other kind of recreational drugs. As such, application of common neuroprotective agents such as BDNF, TMP-1, *etc.* in these cases can be highly desirable. Additionally, immune competence by drug abuse must be prevented by applying anti-addiction agents in the therapeutical regimens. In this context, magnetic nanoformulation of morphine antagonist showed protection of neuronal plasticity during morphine exposure and morphine-treated HIV infection [59]. Similarly, magnetic nanoformulations of other anti-addiction agents can be developed with the aim to prevent deleterious effect in drug addicted HIV patients. Fig. (5) depicts the *in vitro* BBB and rodent model for experimenting ARV transendothelial migration to the brain.

CONTROLLED RELEASE MAGNETIC NANOFORMULATIONS FOR NEUROAIDS

Drug release from aforementioned magnetic nanocarriers remains undefined till date. It is believed that, in an uncontrolled fashion, drug release is mediated by the disease-condition associated modulations of intrinsic cellular phenomenon such as a change in temperature, pH, intracellular Ca^{2+} concentrations, *etc*. Thus, uncertainty persists that if and when drugs are released from magnetic nanocarriers. Approaches are being strategized to develop externally controlled, unambiguous release methods. Recently, novel magneto-electric nanoparticles (MENPs) were developed by fusing $BaTiO_3$ on the $CoFe_2O_4$ core. This multiferroic material possesses strong coupling ability of its magnetic and electric fields at body temperature. The intrinsic high magnetic moment of MENPs can be utilized for their controlled movement under the influence of external, direct current magnetic field, and therefore, effective transendothelial migration of these particles can be achieved. Nonetheless, unlike MNPs, MENPs inherently possess nonzero electric property *i.e.* they respond to alternating current (AC) trigger. Influence of AC trigger can disturb the symmetry of original charge distribution on the surface. Above a certain threshold value of AC field, change in charge distribution can break the ionic bonds between the drugs and nanocarriers leading to controlled drug release phenomenon (Fig. **6A**). Thus both drug delivery and release process from MENPs nanocarriers can be manually controlled from the exterior. MENPs have been used to deliver higher AZTTP concentration across *in vitro* BBB. In this case, application of neither DC field nor AC field modulated the BBB integrity and drug efficacy in suppressing HIV infection was equivalent to that of free drugs as well [66, 67]. Recently MENPs were used to deliver siRNA targeting Beclin1 with the purpose to attenuate the neurotoxic effects of HIV-1 infection in the CNS. The nanoformulation could silence the Beclin1 resulting in significant reduction of viral replication and associated inflammation in brain microglia [68]. An MENPs based formulation was applied to attenuate the effect of cocaine during HIV infection in brain cells. In this case, the therapeutic agent was a microRNA mimic [69]. The integrity of the BBB model remains uncompromised in all these cases.

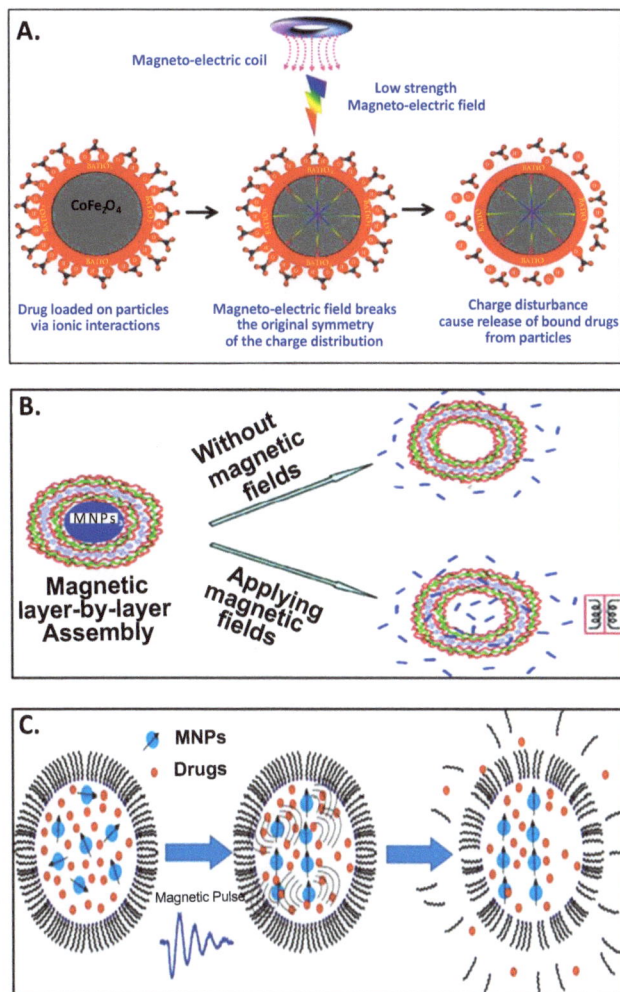

Fig. (6). Mechanisms of controlled drug release from magnetic nanocarriers: (**A**) Application of magneto-electric alternating current (AC) triggers uniform dipole moment in magneto-electric nanoparticles (MENPs). When moment reaches beyond threshold value it disturbs the original charge distribution of surface and subsequently, ionic bonding between MENPs and drugs weakens with the eventual release of drugs [10, 66]. (Reprinted with permission from {Sagar V, Pilakka-Kanthikeel S, Pottathil R, *et al.* Towards nanomedicines for neuroAIDS. Rev. Med. Virol. 2014;24:103–124}, Copyright {2014} the John Wiley and Sons, Ltd.). (**B**) MNPs based layer-by-layer assembly can be disturbed by applying magnetic field-mediated torque which can release drugs from the nanocarriers. Nonetheless, the biodegradable layer-by-layer assembly can also self-degrade over a specific period of time leading to sustained drug release. (Reprinted with permission from {Lu Z, Prouty MD, Quo Z, *et al.* Magnetic switch of permeability for polyelectrolyte microcapsules embedded with Co@Aunanoparticles. Langmuir. 2005;21:2042–2050} [72], Copyright {2005} American Chemical Society). (**C**) Also, the appropriate magnetic pulse can distort the integrity and subsequent permeability of encapsulating materials leading to release of drugs. (Reprinted with permission from {Podaru G, Ogden S, Baxter A, *et al.* Pulsed magnetic field induced fast drug release from magneto-liposomes *via* ultrasound generation. J. Phys. Chem. B. 2014;118:11715–11722} [73], copyright {2014} American Chemical Society).

While electro-responsive ability is one way to control the drug release process, several other stimuli can be fused with magnetic nanoparticles in one or other way. Sagar *et al.* recently showed the ability of MNPs to respond in the presence of transient near infrared exposure and their potential for brain targeting is quite promising [70]. Application of mechanical force by external magnetic field-mediated torque (Fig. **6B**) and magnetic pulse (Fig. **6C**) seems promising as well. Magnetic particles can be also be engineered or coated with those materials which are sensitive to pH, redox, enzymes, glucose, *etc.* and consequently stimuli specific controlled drug release can be achieved [71].

CHALLENGES AND PROSPECTS OF MAGNETIC NANOFORMULATIONS FOR NEUROAIDS

All aforementioned magnetic nanoformulations have shown tremendous promise for targeting HIV sanctuaries in the brain. Proposed mechanism for magnetic nanocarriers based delivery of the drug in the brain is depicted in Fig. (**7**). Nonetheless, their application has not been extended beyond the preclinical laboratory settings. It is highly desirable to identify all associated shortcomings of these nanoformulations so that relevant research can be planned to achieve adequate "*in vitro::in vivo*" correlation [74]. This can open the path to determine nanoformulation's efficacy for clinical success. Major challenges of magnetic nanoformulations are as follows:

1. Loading and bioavailability of bioactive agents: Incorporation of therapeutic agents into magnetic nanocarriers is a most common step and is equally challenging. Fe_3O_4/Fe_2O_3 based nanoparticles possess inverse spinel cubic crystal lattice structures. The face-centered cubic lattices of this structure are occupied by O_{2-} anions. Fe_{2+} or Fe_{3+} anions are occupied at tetrahedral and octahedral sites. Fe moieties at octahedral sites are exposed to environment interfaces. In the aqueous medium, an association of octahedral Fe with OH group cause protonation (Fe-OH+H+ = Fe-OH2+) and deportation (Fe-OH= Fe-O−+H+) (Fig. **3**). Thus depending on the pH of the medium, the positive or negative charge can be generated on the surface of magnetic nanocarriers [54, 75] and this can be used for binding of bioactive agents *via* ionic interaction. Nonetheless, at physiological pH, Fe_3O_4/Fe_2O_3 nanoparticles acquire negative charge [59]. Since not all bioactive agents possess positive charge at physiological pH, their interactions with MNPs is possible by modifying the surface charge using different surfactants or tethering agents. Thus, depending upon the charge pattern of bioactive agents, attention should be given about the tunability in the surface charge of MNPs to achieve maximum drug-nanoparticles binding. Moreover, drug entrapment efficiency can be improved by encapsulation of MNPs in liposomes. Here again determining a successful

incorporation strategy in liposomes is essential to achieve efficient entrapment of drugs and MNPs and this can be achieved by understanding the physicochemical characteristics of liposomes and drugs. Recently, packaging of magnetoliposomes in monocytes/macrophage cells (Fig. **4D**) received significant attention because these cells can naturally reach to the sites of inflammation. Packaged magnetoliposomes in cells serves as the "trojan magnetic nano-vehicle. Importantly, both magnetoliposomes and cell-based carriers prevent drugs bound to nanocarriers from peripheral enzymatic and hydrolytic degradations and thus, drug bioavailability is increased [10, 57]. Influence of magnetic field in driving these nanocarriers to the target in complex physiological setup need intensive investigations. Moreover, a fusion of MNPs with novel materials such as hydrogels should be considered as well. The resulting magnetic nanogels can be beneficial in achieving higher drug load and can prevent drug degradation as well.

2. Biomolecular corona effect: Nanocarriers in peripheral circulation absorb different components of physiological fluid on its surface. This natural functionalization of nanocarriers leads to deposition of different serum factors such as lipids, albumin, immunoglobulin, fibrinogen, complement factors, apolipoproteins, *etc*. Thus, a complex surface layer is formed on nanocarrier's surroundings which are termed as "biomolecular corona". The corona is compartmentalized into hard and soft corona where hard corona molecules have a strong binding affinity to nanocarriers and are deposited on the inner side of the corona. Soft corona molecules are primarily on the outer layers of corona and can be exchanged frequently with the environment. Biomolecular corona formation on drug carriers significantly modulates the biological fate, biodistribution, release, and cellular localization of bound drugs. Even the innate behavior of nanocarriers can acquire unconventional characteristics and therefore pre-designed stimuli condition of nanocarriers may not be functional due to corona effect. Since corona effect is anticipated to have a negative effect on drug delivery and release rate, the inclusion of corona-denaturing agent in the nanocarriers during fabrication can be beneficial. Additionally, nanocarrier's surface can be designed or modified with specific chemicals that can prevent corona formation in entirety [76 - 78]. Thus, corona effect must be taken into consideration during designing a drug carrier so that natural outcome of nanocarriers at a specific target can be achieved.

3. Nanotoxicology and *in vivo* bioavailability: Since the composition of each formulation possesses novelty of one or other kind, their physicochemical characteristics may adversely affect the biological systems. Therefore, it is imperative to evaluate toxicological issues of any xenobiotic before their real-time application. The toxicological evaluation must be extended beyond commonly used cytotoxicity assay to genotoxicity and ecotoxicity as well. The

focus should be directed toward nanomaterials mediated oxidative damage to the cell membrane, DNA and mitochondrial damage, loss of ATP production and uneven gene expression, production of reactive oxygen species and radicals, *etc*. Several approaches may be acquired to mitigate these toxicological effects. In many cases, nanocarriers are functionalized with the biodegradable moieties to nullify the potential toxic effect. Efforts are also being taken to design smart nanocarriers whose degradation can be controlled by specific stimuli after the purpose of nanocarrier is achieved at targeted sites [77]. As stated above, the size of nanocarriers is important in exerting an adverse or positive impact. The adverse effect of MNPs can be minimized by reducing its size to suit hepatobiliary or renal clearance. Nonetheless, MNPs deposition in different body organ must be evaluated because the only permissible limit has non-significant safety concerns. MNPs accumulation in brain peaks between 15 -120 min of exposure of magnetic field which had the intensity of ~1000 Oe. This accumulation in the brain gradually vanishes within 2-3 weeks by unknown mechanisms and it showed no negative physiological effects in mouse [79]. Similarly, MENPs delivery in the brain did not show the sign of neurotoxicity and mouse showed stable neuro-behavioral brain motor coordination activity [80, 81]. Application of biologically produced MNPs can serve as a replacement to counter the toxicological potential of laboratory-made MNPs. It is predicted that nanosized magnetosomes from magnetotactic bacteria can be highly biocompatible [82]. Despite all these limitations, as stated earlier, acceleration of developing MNPs based therapeutics for neuroAIDS will highly depend on an appropriate humanized rodent model and efforts in this direction are intensively applied [35].

4. Limitations of ARV drugs: Current forms of existing drug's carrier require significant engineering transformation to be developed as an ideal carrier for brain targeting. However, beyond the carrier development, neuroAIDS treatments require a strategical shift in applying current ARV drugs and discovery of more effective new drugs. We have already discussed that ARVs can only prevent the HIV infection, and therefore, inclusion of neuron-resuscitating and anti-inflammatory agents in the treatment regimen of neuroAIDS may greatly benefit the survival, development, and function of neurons during HIV infection. Since HIV strains are continuously evolving with new genetic makeup [83], identification of unique strain in each infection case is highly desirable. In fact, approach to target HIV at genomic level, such as HIV genome targeting CRISPR technology [84 - 86] must be the focus of the next generation HIV medicine. Furthermore, designing of novel drugs with the ability to penetrate BBB can greatly help in reducing the menace of HIV and neuroAIDS.

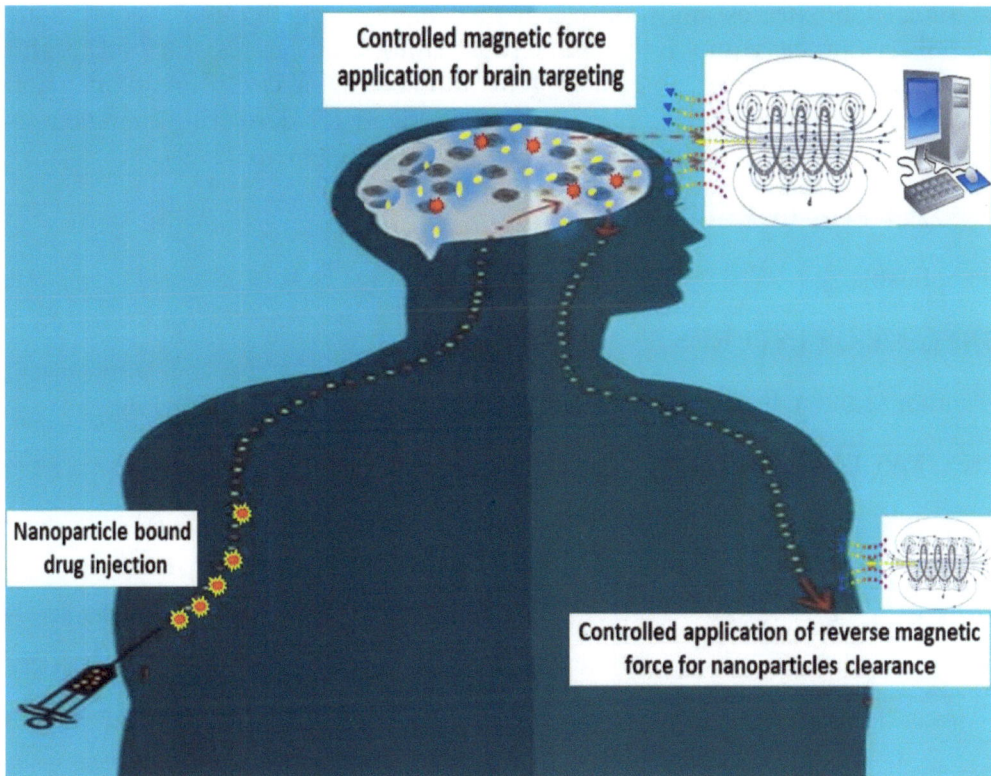

Fig. (7). Depiction of proposed mechanism for magnetic nanocarriers based delivery of the drug in the brain: Nanocarriers can be directed to the brain using in silico-controlled, non-invasive magnetic force from the exterior. Drug release can be controlled using magnetic torque, magnetic pulse, radio-frequency magnetic force, external AC field, *etc.* or natural release can occur due to cellular physicochemical process such as such as a change in temperature, pH, intracellular Ca^{2+}, *etc.* Studies show self-clearance or biodegradation of MNPs in 2-4 weeks. Nonetheless, MNPs can be cleared by applying reverse magnetic force [18]. (BioMed Central allows re-use of content in any way, subject only to proper attribution).

CONCLUSION

Actuation of MNPs using external magnetic force possesses advantages over other existing nanocarriers when it comes to brain targeting. Nonetheless, MNPs application for brain targeting is at crucial juncture because most biomedical applications have been revolving around conventional concepts with only slight modifications in approach. Thus, in order to achieve clinically useful outcomes, it is imperative to look for unconventional ideas which are beyond the current box of nanotechnology. Last six decades of drug delivery technology have swiftly progressed from conventional formulation to smart drug delivery systems [87]. In fact, MNPs have been one of the central components of several smart nanocarrier systems. Application of these nanocarriers for neuroAIDS is currently limited to pre-clinical laboratories study only and they have to go through a continuous evolutionary process involving numerous trials and errors for successful implementation. Moreover, since next-generation medicine is shifting to precision medicine, magnetic nanocarriers must be modulated for delivering therapeutics which can exert desired temporal/permanent changes at genetic levels.

CONSENT FOR PUBLICATION

Not applicable.

CONFLICT OF INTEREST

The author (editor) declares no conflict of interest, financial or otherwise.

ACKNOWLEDGEMENTS

This work was supported in part by grants R01DA040537, R01DA037838, and R01DA034547 from the National Institutes of Health.

REFERENCES

[1]   Letendre SL, Ellis RJ, Everall I, Ances B, Bharti A, McCutchan JA. Neurologic complications of HIV disease and their treatment. Top HIV Med 2009; 17(2): 46-56.
        [PMID: 19401607]

[2]   Nair M, Jayant RD, Kaushik A, Sagar V. Getting into the brain: Potential of nanotechnology in the management of NeuroAIDS. Adv Drug Deliv Rev 2016; 103: 202-17.
        [http://dx.doi.org/10.1016/j.addr.2016.02.008] [PMID: 26944096]

[3]   McArthur JC, Brew BJ, Nath A. Neurological complications of HIV infection. Lancet Neurol 2005; 4(9): 543-55.
        [http://dx.doi.org/10.1016/S1474-4422(05)70165-4] [PMID: 16109361]

[4]   de Almeida SM, Letendre S, Ellis R. Human immunodeficiency virus and the central nervous system. Braz J Infect Dis 2006; 10(1): 41-50.
        [http://dx.doi.org/10.1590/S1413-86702006000100009] [PMID: 16767315]

[5]   McArthur JC. HIV dementia: an evolving disease. J Neuroimmunol 2004; 157(1-2): 3-10.
        [http://dx.doi.org/10.1016/j.jneuroim.2004.08.042] [PMID: 15579274]

[6]   McArthur JC, Haughey N, Gartner S, et al. Human immunodeficiency virus-associated dementia: an evolving disease. J Neurovirol 2003; 9(2): 205-21.
        [http://dx.doi.org/10.1080/13550280390194109] [PMID: 12707851]

[7]   González-Scarano F, Martín-García J. The neuropathogenesis of AIDS. Nat Rev Immunol 2005; 5(1): 69-81.
        [http://dx.doi.org/10.1038/nri1527] [PMID: 15630430]

[8]   Singer EJ, Valdes-Sueiras M, Commins D, et al. Neurologic Presentations of AIDS. Neurol Clin 2010; 28: 253-75.
        [http://dx.doi.org/10.1016/j.ncl.2009.09.018]

[9]   Kramer-Hämmerle S, Rothenaigner I, Wolff H, et al. Cells of the central nervous system as targets and reservoirs of the human immunodeficiency virus. Virus Res 2005; 111: 194-213.

[http://dx.doi.org/10.1016/j.virusres.2005.04.009]

[10]   Sagar V, Pilakka-Kanthikeel S, Pottathil R, Saxena SK, Nair M. Towards nanomedicines for neuroAIDS. Rev Med Virol 2014; 24(2): 103-24.
[http://dx.doi.org/10.1002/rmv.1778] [PMID: 24395761]

[11]   Burdo TH, Lackner A, Williams KC. Monocyte/macrophages and their role in HIV neuropathogenesis. Immunol Rev 2013; 254(1): 102-13.
[http://dx.doi.org/10.1111/imr.12068] [PMID: 23772617]

[12]   Boven LA, Middel J, Breij EC, *et al.* Interactions between HIV-infected monocyte-derived macrophages and human brain microvascular endothelial cells result in increased expression of CC chemokines. J Neurovirol 2000; 6(5): 382-9.
[http://dx.doi.org/10.3109/13550280009018302] [PMID: 11031691]

[13]   Conant K, McArthur JC, Griffin DE, Sjulson L, Wahl LM, Irani DN. Cerebrospinal fluid levels of MMP-2, 7, and 9 are elevated in association with human immunodeficiency virus dementia. Ann Neurol 1999; 46(3): 391-8.
[http://dx.doi.org/10.1002/1531-8249(199909)46:3<391::AID-ANA15>3.0.CO;2-0]   [PMID: 10482270]

[14]   Sporer B, Paul R, Koedel U, *et al.* Presence of matrix metalloproteinase-9 activity in the cerebrospinal fluid of human immunodeficiency virus-infected patients. J Infect Dis 1998; 178(3): 854-7.
[http://dx.doi.org/10.1086/515342] [PMID: 9728558]

[15]   Atluri VS, Hidalgo M, Samikkannu T, *et al.* Effect of human immunodeficiency virus on blood-brain barrier integrity and function: an update. Front Cell Neurosci 2015; 9: 212.
[http://dx.doi.org/10.3389/fncel.2015.00212] [PMID: 26113810]

[16]   Lindl KA, Marks DR, Kolson DL, Jordan-Sciutto KL. HIV-associated neurocognitive disorder: pathogenesis and therapeutic opportunities. J Neuroimmune Pharmacol 2010; 5(3): 294-309.
[http://dx.doi.org/10.1007/s11481-010-9205-z] [PMID: 20396973]

[17]   Nair M, Sagar V, Pilakka-Kanthikeel S. Gene-expression reversal of lncRNAs and associated mRNAs expression in active *vs.* latent HIV infection. Sci Rep 2016; 6: 34862.
[http://dx.doi.org/10.1038/srep34862] [PMID: 27756902]

[18]   Sagar V, Atluri VS, Pilakka-Kanthikeel S, Nair M. Magnetic nanotherapeutics for dysregulated synaptic plasticity during neuroAIDS and drug abuse. Mol Brain 2016; 9(1): 57.
[http://dx.doi.org/10.1186/s13041-016-0236-0] [PMID: 27216740]

[19]   Samikkannu T, Atluri VS, Arias AY, *et al.* HIV-1 subtypes B and C Tat differentially impact synaptic plasticity expression and implicates HIV-associated neurocognitive disorders. Curr HIV Res 2014; 12(6): 397-405.
[http://dx.doi.org/10.2174/1570162X13666150121104720] [PMID: 25613138]

[20]   Atluri VS, Kanthikeel SP, Reddy PV, Yndart A, Nair MP. Human synaptic plasticity gene expression profile and dendritic spine density changes in HIV-infected human CNS cells: role in HIV-associated neurocognitive disorders (HAND). PLoS One 2013; 8(4): e61399.
[http://dx.doi.org/10.1371/journal.pone.0061399] [PMID: 23620748]

[21]   Atluri VS, Pilakka-Kanthikeel S, Samikkannu T, *et al.* Vorinostat positively regulates synaptic plasticity genes expression and spine density in HIV infected neurons: role of nicotine in progression of HIV-associated neurocognitive disorder. Mol Brain 2014; 7: 37.
[http://dx.doi.org/10.1186/1756-6606-7-37] [PMID: 24886748]

[22]   Avdoshina V, Bachis A, Mocchetti I. Synaptic dysfunction in human immunodeficiency virus type--positive subjects: inflammation or impaired neuronal plasticity? J Intern Med 2013; 273(5): 454-65.
[http://dx.doi.org/10.1111/joim.12050] [PMID: 23600400]

[23]   Johanson CE, Stopa EG, McMillan PN. The blood-cerebrospinal fluid barrier: structure and functional significance. Methods Mol Biol 2011; 686: 101-31.

[24] McGee B, Smith N, Aweeka F. HIV pharmacology: barriers to the eradication of HIV from the CNS. HIV Clin Trials 2006; 7(3): 142-53.
[http://dx.doi.org/10.1310/AW2H-TP5C-NP43-K6BY] [PMID: 16880170]

[25] Zhang Z, McGoron AJ, Crumpler ET, Li CZ. Co-culture based blood-brain barrier *in vitro* model, a tissue engineering approach using immortalized cell lines for drug transport study. Appl Biochem Biotechnol 2011; 163(2): 278-95.
[http://dx.doi.org/10.1007/s12010-010-9037-6] [PMID: 20652765]

[26] Wong HL, Wu XY, Bendayan R. Nanotechnological advances for the delivery of CNS therapeutics. Adv Drug Deliv Rev 2012; 64(7): 686-700.
[http://dx.doi.org/10.1016/j.addr.2011.10.007] [PMID: 22100125]

[27] Pardridge WM. Blood-brain barrier drug targeting: the future of brain drug development. Mol Interv 2003; 3: 90-105, 51.
[http://dx.doi.org/10.1124/mi.3.2.90]

[28] Pardridge WM. Alzheimer's disease drug development and the problem of the blood-brain barrier. Alzheimers Dement 2009; 5(5): 427-32.
[http://dx.doi.org/10.1016/j.jalz.2009.06.003] [PMID: 19751922]

[29] Ronaldson PT, Persidsky Y, Bendayan R. Regulation of ABC membrane transporters in glial cells: relevance to the pharmacotherapy of brain HIV-1 infection. Glia 2008; 56(16): 1711-35.
[http://dx.doi.org/10.1002/glia.20725] [PMID: 18649402]

[30] Miller DS. Regulation of P-glycoprotein and other ABC drug transporters at the blood-brain barrier. Trends Pharmacol Sci 2010; 31(6): 246-54.
[http://dx.doi.org/10.1016/j.tips.2010.03.003] [PMID: 20417575]

[31] Wong HL, Chattopadhyay N, Wu XY, *et al.* Nanotechnology applications for improved delivery of antiretroviral drugs to the brain. Adv Drug Deliv Rev 2010; 62: 503-17.
[http://dx.doi.org/10.1016/j.addr.2009.11.020]

[32] Williams R, Bokhari S, Silverstein P, Pinson D, Kumar A, Buch S. Nonhuman primate models of NeuroAIDS. J Neurovirol 2008; 14(4): 292-300.
[http://dx.doi.org/10.1080/13550280802074539] [PMID: 18780230]

[33] Naik P, Cucullo L. *In vitro* blood-brain barrier models: current and perspective technologies. J Pharm Sci 2012; 101(4): 1337-54.
[http://dx.doi.org/10.1002/jps.23022] [PMID: 22213383]

[34] Wilhelm I, Krizbai IA. *In vitro* models of the blood-brain barrier for the study of drug delivery to the brain. Mol Pharm 2014; 11(7): 1949-63.
[http://dx.doi.org/10.1021/mp500046f] [PMID: 24641309]

[35] Jaeger LB, Nath A. Modeling HIV-associated neurocognitive disorders in mice: new approaches in the changing face of HIV neuropathogenesis. Dis. Model. & Mech. Available at: http://dmm.biologists.org/content/5/3/313.abstract 2012.

[36] Evans DT, Silvestri G. Nonhuman primate models in AIDS research. Curr Opin HIV AIDS 2013; 8(4): 255-61.
[PMID: 23615116]

[37] van der Sandt IC, Vos CM, Nabulsi L, *et al.* Assessment of active transport of HIV protease inhibitors in various cell lines and the *in vitro* blood--brain barrier. AIDS 2001; 15(4): 483-91.
[http://dx.doi.org/10.1097/00002030-200103090-00007] [PMID: 11242145]

[38] Park S, Sinko PJ. P-glycoprotein and mutlidrug resistance-associated proteins limit the brain uptake of saquinavir in mice. J Pharmacol Exp Ther 2005; 312(3): 1249-56.
[http://dx.doi.org/10.1124/jpet.104.076216] [PMID: 15528451]

[39] Sun H, Dai H, Shaik N, Elmquist WF. Drug efflux transporters in the CNS. Adv Drug Deliv Rev

2003; 55(1): 83-105.
[http://dx.doi.org/10.1016/S0169-409X(02)00172-2] [PMID: 12535575]

[40]   Sax PE, Wohl D, Yin MT, *et al.* GS-US-292-0104/0111 Study Team. Tenofovir alafenamide *versus* tenofovir disoproxil fumarate, coformulated with elvitegravir, cobicistat, and emtricitabine, for initial treatment of HIV-1 infection: two randomised, double-blind, phase 3, non-inferiority trials. Lancet 2015; 385(9987): 2606-15.
[http://dx.doi.org/10.1016/S0140-6736(15)60616-X] [PMID: 25890673]

[41]   Anderson BD, Morgan ME, Singhal D. Enhanced oral bioavailability of DDI after administration of 6-Cl-ddP, an adenosine deaminase-activated prodrug, to chronically catheterized rats. Pharm Res 1995; 12(8): 1126-33.
[http://dx.doi.org/10.1023/A:1016299507382] [PMID: 7494823]

[42]   Palombo MS, Singh Y, Sinko PJ. Prodrug and conjugate drug delivery strategies for improving HIV/AIDS therapy. J Drug Deliv Sci Technol 2009; 19: 3-14.

[43]   Meairs S, Alonso A. Ultrasound, microbubbles and the blood-brain barrier. Prog Biophys Mol Biol 2007; 93(1-3): 354-62.
[http://dx.doi.org/10.1016/j.pbiomolbio.2006.07.019] [PMID: 16959303]

[44]   Burgess A, Shah K, Hough O, Hynynen K. Focused ultrasound-mediated drug delivery through the blood-brain barrier. Expert Rev Neurother 2015; 15(5): 477-91.
[http://dx.doi.org/10.1586/14737175.2015.1028369] [PMID: 25936845]

[45]   Salahuddin TS, Johansson BB, Kalimo H, Olsson Y. Structural changes in the rat brain after carotid infusions of hyperosmolar solutions. An electron microscopic study. Acta Neuropathol 1988; 77(1): 5-13.
[http://dx.doi.org/10.1007/BF00688236] [PMID: 3149121]

[46]   Fleegal-DeMotta MA, Doghu S, Banks WA. Angiotensin II modulates BBB permeability *via* activation of the AT(1) receptor in brain endothelial cells. J Cereb Blood Flow Metab 2009; 29(3): 640-7.
[http://dx.doi.org/10.1038/jcbfm.2008.158] [PMID: 19127280]

[47]   Sood RR, Taheri S, Candelario-Jalil E, Estrada EY, Rosenberg GA. Early beneficial effect of matrix metalloproteinase inhibition on blood-brain barrier permeability as measured by magnetic resonance imaging countered by impaired long-term recovery after stroke in rat brain. J Cereb Blood Flow Metab 2008; 28(2): 431-8.
[http://dx.doi.org/10.1038/sj.jcbfm.9600534] [PMID: 17700631]

[48]   Qin LJ, Gu YT, Zhang H, Xue YX. Bradykinin-induced blood-tumor barrier opening is mediated by tumor necrosis factor-α. Neurosci Lett 2009; 450(2): 172-5.
[http://dx.doi.org/10.1016/j.neulet.2008.10.080] [PMID: 18983897]

[49]   Gunaseelan S, Gunaseelan K, Deshmukh M, Zhang X, Sinko PJ. Surface modifications of nanocarriers for effective intracellular delivery of anti-HIV drugs. Adv Drug Deliv Rev 2010; 62(4-5): 518-31.
[http://dx.doi.org/10.1016/j.addr.2009.11.021] [PMID: 19941919]

[50]   Roy U, McMillan J, Alnouti Y, *et al.* Pharmacodynamic and antiretroviral activities of combination nanoformulated antiretrovirals in HIV-1-infected human peripheral blood lymphocyte-reconstituted mice. J Infect Dis 2012; 206(10): 1577-88.
[http://dx.doi.org/10.1093/infdis/jis395] [PMID: 22811299]

[51]   Gupta U, Jain NK. Non-polymeric nano-carriers in HIV/AIDS drug delivery and targeting. Adv Drug Deliv Rev 2010; 62: 478-90.

[52]   Pan Y, Du X, Zhao F, Xu B. Magnetic nanoparticles for the manipulation of proteins and cells. Chem Soc Rev 2012; 41(7): 2912-42.
[http://dx.doi.org/10.1039/c2cs15315g] [PMID: 22318454]

[53]   Chaughule RS, Purushotham S, Ramanujan RV. Magnetic Nanoparticles as Contrast Agents for

Magnetic Resonance Imaging. Proc. Natl. Acad. Sci. India Sect. A Phys. Sci [Internet] 2012; 82: 257-68.
[http://dx.doi.org/10.1007/s40010-012-0038-4]

[54]   Tombacz E. Magnetite in aqueous medium: coating its surface and surface coated with it. Rom Rep Phys 2006; 58: 281-6.

[55]   Ding H, Sagar V, Agudelo M, *et al.* Enhanced blood-brain barrier transmigration using a novel transferrin embedded fluorescent magneto-liposome nanoformulation. Nanotechnology 2014; 25(5): 055101.
[http://dx.doi.org/10.1088/0957-4484/25/5/055101] [PMID: 24406534]

[56]   Saiyed ZM, Gandhi NH, Nair MP. Magnetic nanoformulation of azidothymidine 5′-triphosphate for targeted delivery across the blood-brain barrier. Int J Nanomedicine 2010; 5: 157-66.
[PMID: 20463931]

[57]   Jain S, Mishra V, Singh P, *et al.* RGD-anchored magnetic liposomes for monocytes/neutrophils-mediated brain targeting. Int J Pharm 2003; 261: 43-55.

[58]   Jain TK, Reddy MK, Morales MA, Leslie-Pelecky DL, Labhasetwar V. Biodistribution, clearance, and biocompatibility of iron oxide magnetic nanoparticles in rats. Mol Pharm 2008; 5(2): 316-27.
[http://dx.doi.org/10.1021/mp7001285] [PMID: 18217714]

[59]   Sagar V, Pilakka-Kanthikeel S, Atluri VS, *et al.* Therapeutical neurotargeting *via* magnetic nanocarrier: Implications to opiate-induced neuropathogenesis and NeuroAIDS. J Biomed Nanotechnol 2015; 11(10): 1722-33.
[http://dx.doi.org/10.1166/jbn.2015.2108] [PMID: 26502636]

[60]   Jayant RD, Atluri VS, Agudelo M, Sagar V, Kaushik A, Nair M. Sustained-release nanoART formulation for the treatment of neuroAIDS. Int J Nanomedicine 2015; 10: 1077-93.
[http://dx.doi.org/10.2147/IJN.S76517] [PMID: 25709433]

[61]   Fiandra L, Colombo M, Mazzucchelli S, *et al.* Nanoformulation of antiretroviral drugs enhances their penetration across the blood brain barrier in mice. Nanomedicine (Lond) 2015; 11(6): 1387-97.
[http://dx.doi.org/10.1016/j.nano.2015.03.009] [PMID: 25839392]

[62]   Wen X, Wang K, Zhao Z, *et al.* Brain-targeted delivery of trans-activating transcriptor-conjugated magnetic PLGA/lipid nanoparticles. PLoS One 2014; 9(9): e106652.
[http://dx.doi.org/10.1371/journal.pone.0106652] [PMID: 25187980]

[63]   Raymond AD, Diaz P, Chevelon S, *et al.* Microglia-derived HIV Nef+ exosome impairment of the blood-brain barrier is treatable by nanomedicine-based delivery of Nef peptides. J Neurovirol 2016; 22(2): 129-39.
[http://dx.doi.org/10.1007/s13365-015-0397-0] [PMID: 26631079]

[64]   Atluri VS, Jayant RD, Pilakka-Kanthikeel S, *et al.* Development of TIMP1 magnetic nanoformulation for regulation of synaptic plasticity in HIV-1 infection. Int J Nanomedicine 2016; 11: 4287-98.
[http://dx.doi.org/10.2147/IJN.S108329] [PMID: 27621622]

[65]   Pilakka-Kanthikeel S, Atluri VS, Sagar V, Saxena SK, Nair M. Targeted brain derived neurotropic factors (BDNF) delivery across the blood-brain barrier for neuro-protection using magnetic nano carriers: an *in vitro* study. PLoS One 2013; 8(4): e62241.
[http://dx.doi.org/10.1371/journal.pone.0062241] [PMID: 23653680]

[66]   Nair M, Guduru R, Liang P, Hong J, Sagar V, Khizroev S. Externally controlled on-demand release of anti-HIV drug using magneto-electric nanoparticles as carriers. Nat Commun 2013; 4: 1707.
[http://dx.doi.org/10.1038/ncomms2717] [PMID: 23591874]

[67]   Kaushik A, Jayant RD, Sagar V, Nair M. The potential of magneto-electric nanocarriers for drug delivery. Expert Opin Drug Deliv 2014; 11(10): 1635-46.
[http://dx.doi.org/10.1517/17425247.2014.933803] [PMID: 24986772]

[68]   Rodriguez M, Kaushik A, Lapierre J, *et al.* Electro-Magnetic Nano-Particle Bound Beclin1 siRNA

Crosses the Blood???Brain Barrier to Attenuate the Inflammatory Effects of HIV-1 Infection *in vitro*. J Neuroimmune Pharmacol 2016; 1-13.
[PMID: 27287620]

[69]   Sagar V, Pilakka-Kanthikeel S, Ding H, Atluri VS, Jayant RD, Kaushik AN. Novel magneto-electric nanodelivery of microRNA mimic across blood-brain barrier: Implications to cocaine modulation on HIV-associated neurocognitive disorders. J Neuroimmune Pharmacol 2014; 9: S49.

[70]   Sagar V, Atluri VS, Tomitaka A, *et al.* Coupling of transient near infrared photonic with magnetic nanoparticle for potential dissipation-free biomedical application in brain. Sci Rep 2016; 6: 29792.
[http://dx.doi.org/10.1038/srep29792] [PMID: 27465276]

[71]   Sagar V, Nair M. Near-infrared biophotonics-based nanodrug release systems and their potential application for neuro-disorders. Expert Opin Drug Deliv 2017; 1-16.
[http://dx.doi.org/10.1080/17425247.2017.1297794] [PMID: 28276967]

[72]   Lu Z, Prouty MD, Guo Z, Golub VO, Kumar CS, Lvov YM. Magnetic switch of permeability for polyelectrolyte microcapsules embedded with Co@Au nanoparticles. Langmuir 2005; 21(5): 2042-50.
[http://dx.doi.org/10.1021/la047629q] [PMID: 15723509]

[73]   Podaru G, Ogden S, Baxter A, *et al.* Pulsed magnetic field induced fast drug release from magneto liposomes *via* ultrasound generation. J Phys Chem B 2014; 118(40): 11715-22.
[http://dx.doi.org/10.1021/jp5022278] [PMID: 25110807]

[74]   Lu Y, Sungwon Kim KP. In vitro-In vivo Correlation : Perspectives on Model Development 2012; 418: 142-8.

[75]   Ghose SK, Petitto SC, Tanwar KS, *et al.* Chapter 1 Surface Structure and Reactivity of Iron Oxide–Water Interfaces. Dev Earth Environ Sci 2007; 7: 1-29.

[76]   Docter D, Westmeier D, Markiewicz M, Stolte S, Knauer SK, Stauber RH. The nanoparticle biomolecule corona: lessons learned - challenge accepted? Chem Soc Rev 2015; 44(17): 6094-121.
[http://dx.doi.org/10.1039/C5CS00217F] [PMID: 26065524]

[77]   Karimi M, Ghasemi A, Sahandi Zangabad P, *et al.* Smart micro/nanoparticles in stimulus-responsive drug/gene delivery systems. Chem Soc Rev 2016; 45(5): 1457-501.

[78]   Lundqvist M, Stigler J, Cedervall T, *et al.* The evolution of the protein corona around nanoparticles: a test study. ACS Nano 2011; 5(9): 7503-9.
[http://dx.doi.org/10.1021/nn202458g] [PMID: 21861491]

[79]   Kong SD, Lee J, Ramachandran S, *et al.* Magnetic targeting of nanoparticles across the intact blood-brain barrier. J Control Release 2012; 164(1): 49-57.
[http://dx.doi.org/10.1016/j.jconrel.2012.09.021] [PMID: 23063548]

[80]   Kaushik A, Jayant RD, Nikkhah-Moshaie R, *et al.* Magnetically guided central nervous system delivery and toxicity evaluation of magneto-electric nanocarriers. Sci Rep 2016; 6: 25309.
[http://dx.doi.org/10.1038/srep25309] [PMID: 27143580]

[81]   Sagar V, Huang Z, Kaushik A, *et al.* Effect of Magneto-electric nanoparticle on deep brain motor coordination activity. J Neuroimmune Pharmacol 2015; 10: S99-S100.

[82]   Sun J, Li Y, Liang XJ, Wang PC. Bacterial magnetosome: A novel biogenetic magnetic targeted drug carrier with potential multifunctions. J Nanomater 2011; 2011(2011): 469031-43.
[PMID: 22448162]

[83]   Kozal MJ. Drug-resistant human immunodefiency virus. Clin Microbiol Infect 2009; 15 (Suppl. 1): 69-73.
[http://dx.doi.org/10.1111/j.1469-0691.2008.02687.x] [PMID: 19220361]

[84]   Wang Z, Pan Q, Gendron P, *et al.* CRISPR/Cas9-derived mutations both inhibit HIV-1 replication and accelerate viral escape. Cell Reports 2016; 15(3): 481-9.
[http://dx.doi.org/10.1016/j.celrep.2016.03.042] [PMID: 27068471]

[85]   Zhu W, Lei R, Le Duff Y, *et al.* The CRISPR/Cas9 system inactivates latent HIV-1 proviral DNA. Retrovirology 2015; 12: 22.
[http://dx.doi.org/10.1186/s12977-015-0150-z] [PMID: 25808449]

[86]   Liang C, Wainberg MA, Das AT, Berkhout B. CRISPR/Cas9: a double-edged sword when used to combat HIV infection. Retrovirology 2016; 13(1): 37.
[http://dx.doi.org/10.1186/s12977-016-0270-0] [PMID: 27230886]

[87]   Yun YH, Lee BK, Park K. Controlled Drug Delivery: Historical perspective for the next generation. J Control Release 2015; 219: 2-7.
[http://dx.doi.org/10.1016/j.jconrel.2015.10.005] [PMID: 26456749]

CHAPTER 3

Syntheses of FDA Approved Integrase Inhibitor HIV Drugs and Improved Manufacturing using Flow Processing

Omobolanle Janet Jesumoroti, Faith Akwi and **Paul Watts**[*]

Nelson Mandela University, University Way, Port Elizabeth, 6031, South Africa

Abstract: A number of new antiviral drugs have made HIV/AIDS a manageable disease by the introduction of integrase strand transfer inhibitors. One of the major concerns is the accessibility of these drugs in lower income countries. Thus, adequate supplies and cost effective syntheses of these drugs *via* flow technology are of great importance. Presently, there are four integrase strand transfer inhibitors approved by FDA. This chapter will focus on the published synthesis of currently FDA approved integrase inhibitor drugs and other HIV drugs developed through flow technology. Thus hoping that such a review could be useful to scientists and academia desiring a greater understanding of HIV integrase drug development at reduced cost and could serve as a context for further research and possible collaboration with the industry.

Keywords: Active pharmaceutical intermediate, Batch synthesis, Continuous flow synthesis, Food and drug administration, HIV/AIDS, HIV integrase, HIV protease, Integrase strand transfer inhibitor, Microreactors, Process development.

INTRODUCTION

Synthetic chemistry involves the development of new synthetic reactions, methods, and strategies of forming new chemical bonds, thus allowing the discovery of more complex pharmaceutical drug candidates [1 - 3]. This has great impact on our society since clinical agents against diseases can be developed through it thus resulting in a steady increase in life expectancy [4]. Despite the advent of highly active antiretroviral therapy (HAARTs) which drastically improved both quality and the length of life of human immunodeficiency virus (HIV)-infected patients [5, 6], over 35 million people have died of Acquired Immunodeficiency Syndrome (AIDS)/HIV related diseases since the start of the

[*] **Corresponding Author Paul Watts:** Nelson Mandela University, University Way, Port Elizabeth, 6031, South Africa; Tel: +27415043694; Fax: +27415049281; Email: Paul.Watts@mandela.ac.za

Atta-ur-Rahman (Ed.)

epidemic. 1.8 million new HIV infections have been reported to occur across the globe yearly [7].

The viral cycle of HIV comprises of seven stages that are considered to be druggable targets: 1). binding (viral adsorption to the cell membrane), 2). fusion between the viral envelope and the cell membrane, 3). reverse transcription of the viral RNA (Ribonucleic Acid) to proviral DNA (Deoxyribonucleic Acid), 4). integration of the viral DNA into the DNA of CD_4 cells, 5). DNA replication, 6). viral assembly and 7). budding and release of new mature virions. Each step in the replicative cycle of HIV is crucial and the majority of chemotherapeutic approaches focused on the development of retroviral enzyme inhibitors are aimed at step 3 (reverse transcription, RT), step 4 (integrase, IN), and step 6 (protease PR) [8]. Step 4 (integrase, IN) is critical for stable HIV-1 infection wherein the integration of HIV DNA into the host cell's chromosomal DNA takes place.

HIV-1 viral replication requires three encoded enzymes: nucleoside protease, reverse transcriptase and integrase. The latter is crucial for the integration of HIV DNA into the host cell chromosomal DNA, a step that is critical for stable HIV-1 infection due to lack of homologous enzymes in a human host [9]. As such, it is a rational target for anti-AIDS therapy. Integration involves two key processes: 3' processing and strand transfer [10]. The integration of the viral DNA into the host chromosome occurs through a series of DNA cutting and joining reactions. The first step involves the removal of two nucleotides from each 3'-end of the viral DNA, a process called 3'-end processing, while the second step, termed as DNA strand transfer involves the processed viral DNA ends covalently joining the host DNA [11]. The currently approved integrase strand transfer inhibitors (INSTIs) block integrase's active site and prevent the pre-integration complex from binding to host DNA thus resulting in inactive non-integrated proviral HIV DNA [11].

The INSTIs, a class of antiretroviral drugs, have become a standard of care in guidelines for first-line therapy in treatment of HIV-1 infection [12]. They offer minimal toxicity, high antiviral potency with rapid decline in HIV RNA. Additionally, they have a relatively low daily dosing plan, favourable clinical and safety profile, good tolerability, lack of significant drug-drug interactions and cross-resistance to other anti-HIV drug classes [13, 14]. To date, there are four INSTIs on the market that have been approved by the Food and Drug Administration (FDA): Raltegravir [approved 2007(RAL)] [15]. Elvitegravir [approved 2012 (EVG)] and Dolutegravir [approved 2013 (DTG)], Bictegravir (2018) while an investigational drug (Carbotegravir) is in phase IIb clinical trial. These drugs share many characteristics including mechanism of action, antiviral potency, good safety and tolerability profile, but differ from each other in terms of formulation, dosing resistance and interactions profile.

Several new antivirals drugs have made HIV a manageable disease however, the cost of treatment is still unaffordable for many patients in lower income countries [16]. As such, there are concerted efforts by researchers and pharmaceutical companies across the world to continuously seek ways to hasten this development process by embracing new synthetic approaches and enabling technologies in order to cost-effectively produce new drugs for both new and old targets [17]. As part of the "Medicines for All" initiative funded by the Bill and Melinda Gates Foundation [18], continuous flow technology seeks cheaper and more efficient ways to manufacture drugs, particularly those needed to treat human immunodeficiency virus (HIV) and acquired immune deficiency syndrome (AIDS) in developing countries [19]. This is attributed to the various benefits it offers to organic chemical syntheses [20 - 22]. At present, a couple of research groups have investigated the continuous flow synthesis of some HIV/AIDS drugs and active pharmaceutical intermediates (APIs) such as Nevirapine [19], Dolutergravir [23], Efavirenz [24, 25], Lamivudine [26], Atazanavir and Darunavir [27, 28]. It is also worth mentioning that a continuous flow process for the manufacture of Darunavir, has already been approved by the FDA and European Medicine Agency [29, 30]. It is of no doubt that continuous flow technology offers tremendous opportunity for the discovery of new process windows in drug and API synthesis.

The aim of this chapter is to provide a comprehensive foundation and reference source for scientists, public health officials, funding organizations, policymakers and academia desiring a greater understanding of the synthesis of HIV drug and APIs development. Herein, we intend to discuss the recent developments in the generic and most scalable batch and flow synthesis routes based on published or patent literature of clinically approved HIV integrase inhibitors and other HIV drugs & APIs over the past decade (2007-2018).

BATCH SYNTHESIS OF FDA APPROVED HIV INTEGRASE INHIBITORS

In this section, we discuss the traditional approach towards the synthesis of HIV strand transfer inhibitors, INSTIs that are currently on the market Fig. (**1**).

RALTEGRAVIR

Background

Raltegravir (RAL) (Isentress) **1** (Fig. 1), produced by Merck & Co as a potassium salt, launched in October 2007 is the first FDA approved integrase (IN) inhibitor. It is a pyrimidine carboxamide integrase inhibitor structurally based on a diketo

acid moiety [15]. Its chemical name is 4-[*N*-(4-fluorobenzyl)carbamoyl-
-1-methyl-2- [1-methyl-1-(5-methyl-1,3,4-oxadiazol-2ylcarboxamido. The β-
hydroxy-ketone structural motif allows blocking of integrase's active site through
interaction with divalent metals within the active site of HIV [31]. Raltegravir **l**
was initially used as combination therapy with other antiretroviral agents for the
treatment of the human immunodeficiency virus (HIV-1) and later as first-line
therapy in ARV-naive patients and pediatric populations [32, 33]. It is
administered orally twice-daily as a tablet of 400 mg strength. It also has good
safety and antiviral activity [34]. A new formulation of Raltegravir: Isentress HD
(high dose), approved in 2017 as part of the treatment of HIV, provides a simpler
and a convenient alternative to the twice-daily Raltegravir tablets as it can be
administered once daily as a tablet of 600 mg strength with or without ingestion
of food [35].

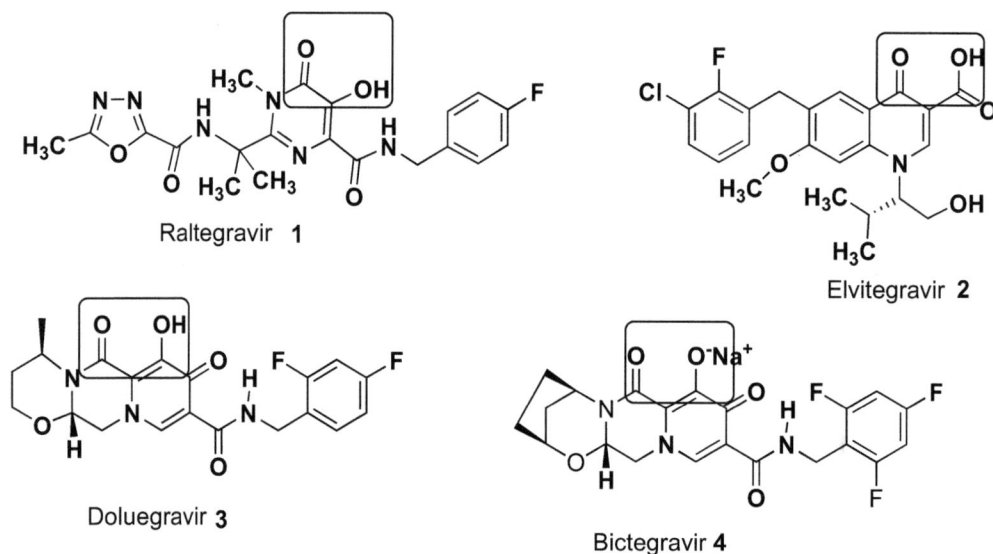

Fig. (1). FDA Approved Integrase Inhibitors.

Synthesis of Raltegravir

Raltegravir **1** can be disconnected into four components; oxadiazole carbonyl
chloride **15**, methyl iodide, 4-fluorobenzylamine (4-FBA) and the densely
functionalized hydroxypyrimidinone **10** (Fig. **2**) due to cleavage of two amide
bonds and a C-N bond. Once these individual fragments are prepared, it is
relatively straightforward to link them together to complete the synthesis of
Raltegravir. A brief discussion of the routes used by the discovery chemists and
the process chemists to deliver multikilogram quantities of Raltegravir **1** are
summarised below.

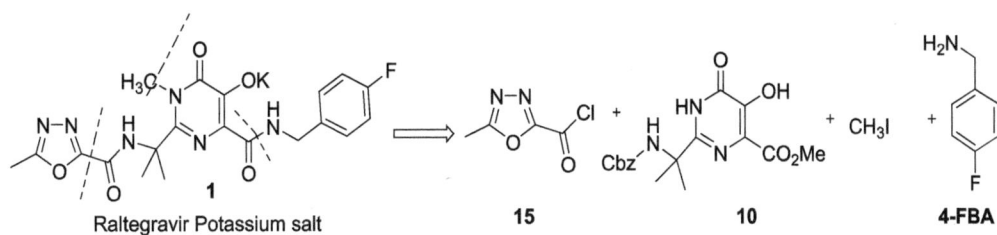

Fig. (2). Retrosynthesis Analysis of Raltegravir [15].

In 2008, Raltegravir **1** was first prepared in 10 linear steps (15) (Scheme **1**) starting from Strecker reaction of commercially available and inexpensive free phenol. In this procedure, the free phenol was converted to 2-amino-2-methylpropanenitrile **6** followed by Cbz protection of aminonitrile **6** under Schotten–Baumann condition to nitrile **7**. Hydroxylamine addition to **7** provided amidoxime **8**.

The subsequent two-component-coupling reaction of **8** with dimethylacetylenedicarboxylate (DMAD) afforded a *Z/E* mixtures of **9** which then cyclised through thermal rearrangement to form dihydroxy-pyrimidine-2-carboxylates **10**. Selective hydroxyl protection (Benzylation) followed by chromatographic purification afforded the 2-substituted methyl 5-(benzoyloxy)-1-methyl-6-oxo-1,6- dihydro-pyrimidine-4-carboxylates **11** with the *O*-methylated pyrimidine analogue as a minor product. *N*-methylation of **11** with methylsulphate using LiH as a base and dioxane followed by another chromatographic purification to remove *O*-methylated impurity afforded intermediate **13**. Hydrogenation of **13** with Pd/C as a catalyst afforded free amine **14** which when amidated with oxadiazole carbonyl chloride **15**, provided intermediate **16** which was then converted into the target compound Raltegravir **1** by amidation with 4-fluorobenzylamine.

However, the discovery route suffers several low yielding steps and serious drawback of removing *O*-methylation and *O*-acylation impurities by several purification processes using either column chromatography or recrystallization thereby reducing the overall yield to 3% and making the process unattractive for industrial use. In addition, the use of highly toxic and expensive dioxane and halogenated solvents such as chloroform, dichloromethane that present an unreasonable risk to health and environment are not desirable for commercial purpose.

In an attempt to develop convenient higher yielding and more environmentally friendly routes on an industrial scale for the synthesis of Raltegravir **1** and its salts, Humphrey *et al.* [36] developed a first generation process synthetic route

(Scheme **2**) that addressed the key chemical, productivity, and environmental impact issues of the initial synthesis of Raltegravir/isentress by Summa *et al.* [15] The author identified the key challenges in the synthesis of Raltegravir **1** were the efficient construction of the hydroxypyrimidinone core **10** and the optimization of the selective *N*-methylation amidoxime. Even though the fundamental disconnection remained the same, modification of reagents and conditions were essential for the successful preparation of Raltegravir **1**. The synthesis of hydroxypyrimidinone core **10** was investigated by first optimizing the synthesis of amidoxine **8** since the yield of hydroxypyrimidinone core **10** depends on the products of *E/Z* configuration of **9**.

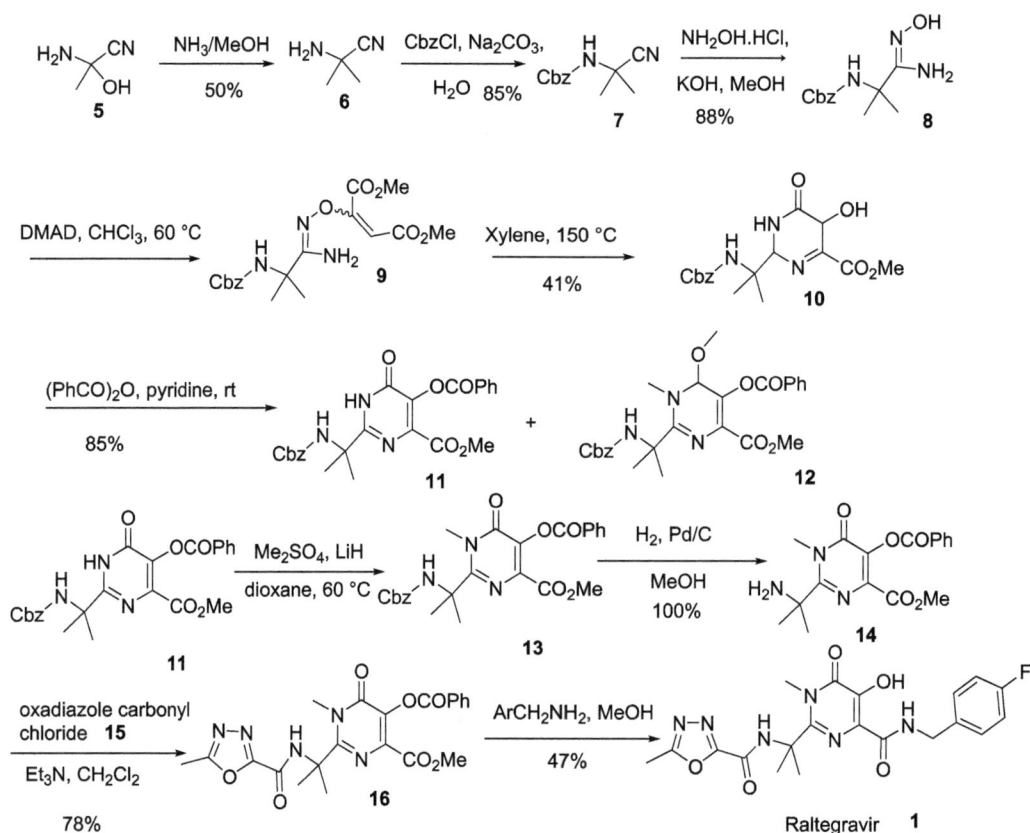

Scheme 1. Synthesis of Raltegravir [15]. Process Development.

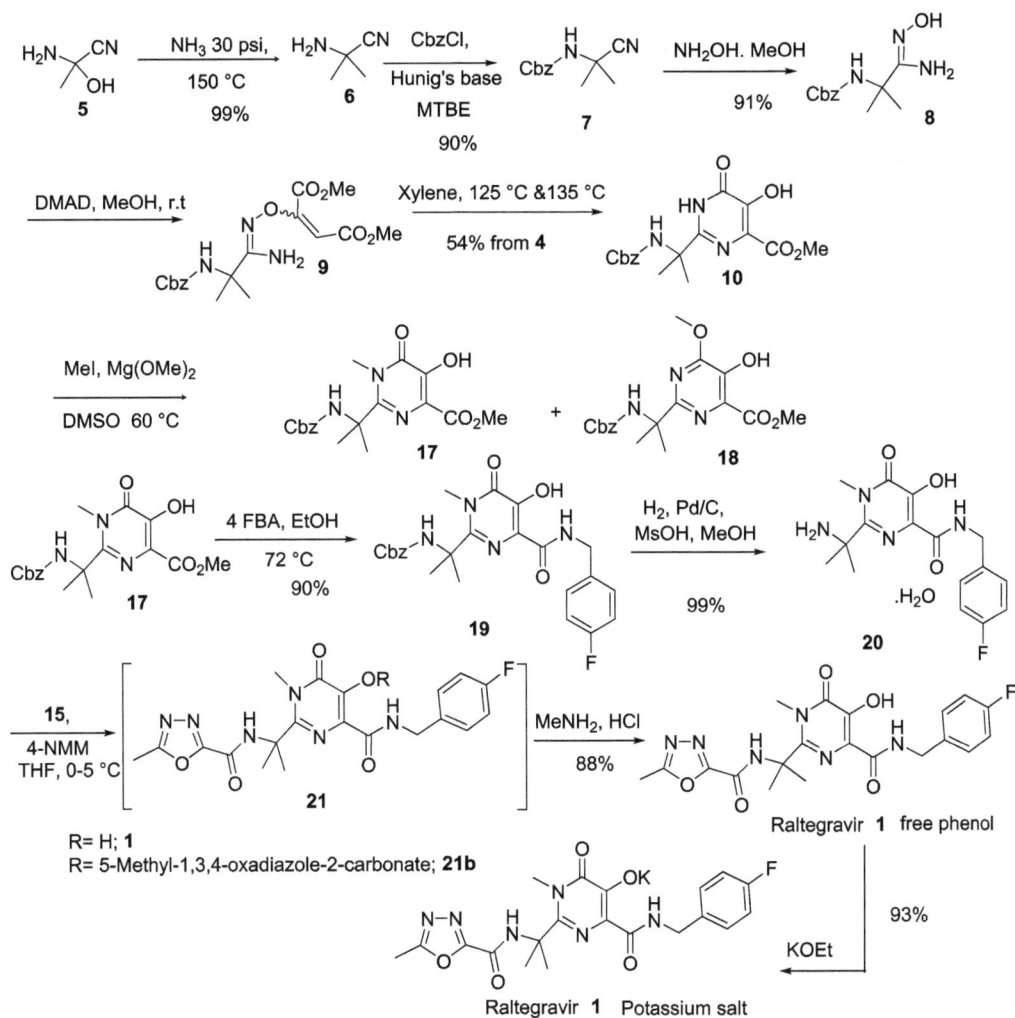

Scheme 2. Synthesis of Raltegravir [36] first generation synthetic route.

As shown Scheme **2** the use of 1.5 equiv of neat liquid ammonia at 30 psi and 150 °C for the Strecker reaction gave a 99% yield. The treatment of aminonitrile **6** with benzyl chloroformate afforded *N*-Cbz-protected intermediate **7** in 90% assay yield. In general, the use of alternative reagents in the synthetic routes of the amidoxine **8** yielded 91% of the desired product. An increase in the overall isolated yield (37% to 81%) over the three reaction steps was observed.

The process synthesis paralleled the discovery route from **5** through **9** to provide **10**, with an improved yield (54%) for the dihydroxypyrimidine **10**. Direct *N*-methylation of **10** with methyl iodide as methylating agent, magnesium methoxide as a base for deprotonation and DMSO as a solvent at 60 °C afforded methylpyrimidone **17** in 78% assay yield and *O*-methylpyrimidine side product. Amidation of **17** with fluorobenzylamide was accomplished by treatment in ethanol at 72 °C followed by crystallization to provide **19** in 90% isolated yield. This was followed by hydrogenation of the Cbz-protected amine **19** with 5% Pd/C and MsOH followed by catalyst filtration and neutralization with NaOH to afford **20** as a hygroscopic hydrated product in 99% isolated yield. **20** required drying before the final oxadiazole coupling. Final installation of the oxadiazole **15** with amine **20** afforded the free hydroxyl form of Raltegravir **1** and the ester **21b**. Treatment of the reaction mixture **21** with MeNH$_2$ cleaves the ester and acidification with HCl, followed by crystallization and filtration afforded the free phenol Raltegravir **1** in 88% isolated yield, which was converted to Raltegravir potassium **1** in 93% yield and 99.5% purity when treated with potassium ethoxide.

Note: The synthesis of the oxadiazole **15** (Scheme **3**) began with the reaction of methyltetrazole **22** with ethyl oxalyl chloride **23** to provide the ethyl oxalyltetrazole intermediate **24** which rearranged with loss of nitrogen on heating in toluene. Saponification of the crude ethyl ester with potassium hydroxide gave the oxadiazole carboxylate salt **15**.

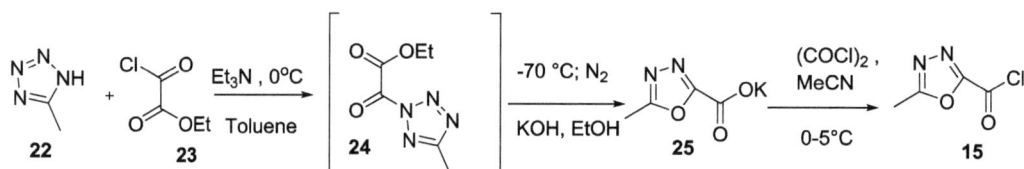

Scheme 3. The Synthesis of the oxadiazole [36].

Many aspects of the first-generation synthesis made it suitable for the large scale preparation of Raltegravir **1**. These include high yielding nine linear steps with 22% overall yield, high efficient construction of the key highly functionalized hydroxypyrimidone **10** in a single step through thermal rearrangement of amidoxime DMAD adducts, elimination of halogenated highly toxic and expensive solvents, substitution of undesired base LiH with Mg(OMe)$_2$ and elimination of chromatographic purification. Nevertheless, the first-generation route relies on the hygroscopic hydrated amine which is difficult to dry, excessive use of expensive 4-FBA (2.3 equiv) and oxadiazole (2.2 equiv), moderate methylation selectivity, low volume productivity and high waste production (PMI). This necessitated the improvement of this route in order to meet global patient access of **1**.

Within the first and second-generation development routes [36], the same cyclo isomerization strategy was used to prepare the key hydroxyl pyrimidinone **10**;

however, the redesigned synthesis was targeted at reversing the order of subsequent steps from **10** to **1**, thereby introducing amide group early in the synthesis before methylation (Scheme **4**).

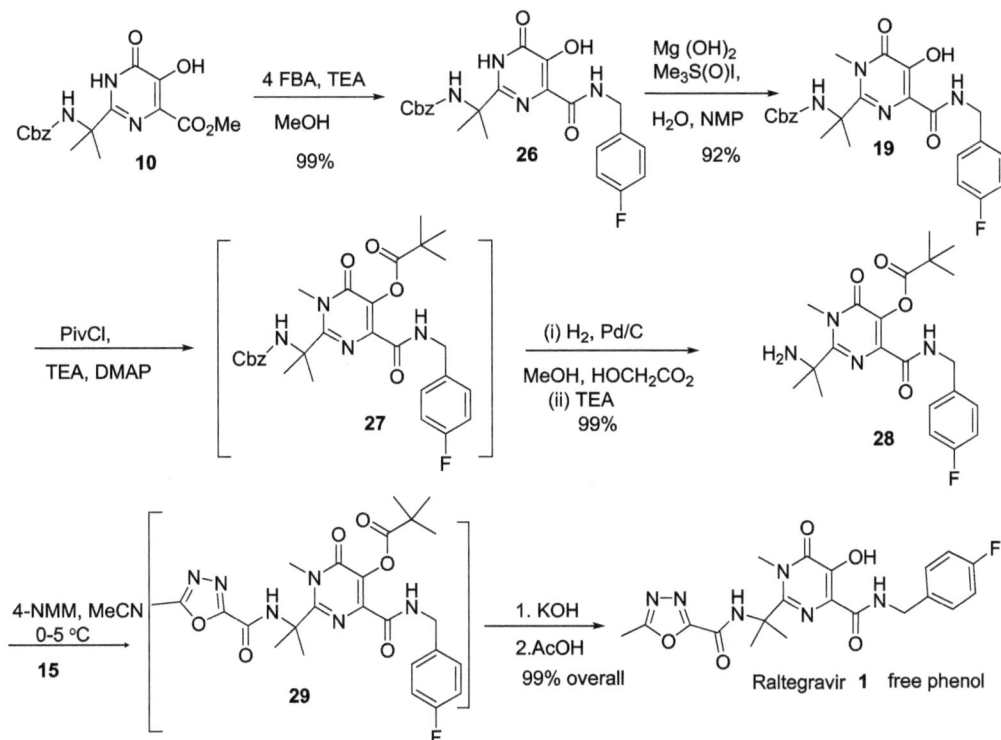

Scheme 4. Synthesis of Raltegravir [36] second generation synthetic route.

Thus, the second generation route starts with the synthesis of key intermediate hydroxyl pyrimidinone **10** by following Humphrey's procedure as shown in Scheme **2**. This was then treated with 1.4 equiv of 4-FBA and 1 equiv of TEA in MeOH to afford **26** which was then methylated with 2 equiv of trimethyl-sulfoxonium iodide $Me_3S(O)I$, 2 equiv of magnesium hydroxide, 1 equiv of $H2O$ and NMP to afford **19**. Acylation of Cbz-amide **26** at room temperature with pivaloyl chloride (PivCl) in the presence of triethylamine and DMAP afforded crude pivalate ester **27**. The treatment of crude **27** with water followed by hydrogenation with Pd/C in the presence of methanol and glycolic acid at 20-25 °C and finally treatment with Net_3 afforded free amine pivalate ester **28** as a non-hygrocopic solid. With the free amine pivalate ester **28** in hand, the synthesis of free phenol **1** was initiated by preparing slurry of **28** using 4-NMM in acetonitrile and coupling it with acyl chloride **15** at -10 °C to afford **29**. Finally, the complete synthesis of free phenol **1** was achieved by the addition of KOH followed by AcOH to **26** in 99% isolated yield.

This process has several advantages: (1). identification of pivalated amine intermediate **28** as a non- hygroscopic solid (2). *In situ* demethylation– remethylation to isomerize the *O*-methyl to the desired *N*-methyl pyrimidinone (3). use of low equivalent of both oxadiazole **15** and 4-FBA, (4). does not employ solvent switches, (5). less complex from a process point of view, and (6). more productive.

The first-generation manufacturing procedure was successfully scaled up to provide multi-tonne quantities of the bulk drug with consistent high purity. The conversion of hydroxyl pyrimidinone **10** to Raltegravir **2** resulted in increase in overall yield from 20% in the original discovery routes to 51% in first generation process route and finally to 84% in the second generation process routes. The highlights of the new synthesis route include 3 to 5-fold higher productivity, a highly selective methylation, and a 65% reduction of combined aqueous and organic waste produced. This new synthetic route provides Raltegravir potassium in 35% overall yield.

Mukund *et al.* [37] reported a more convenient process synthetic route for the preparation of Isentress/Raltegravir **1** and its salts. The author disclosed the invention to be a cost effective process with fewer synthetic steps thus limiting formation of impurities and therefore making it environmentally friendly and more attractive for industrial scale. The synthetic protocols avoid the use of protection and deprotection of the amine group as described in the second-generation process methods.

The synthesis shown in Scheme **5** involved the reaction between 2-amino-2-methylpropanenitrile **6** with oxadiazole carbonyl chloride **15** to give *N*-(2-cyanopropan-2-yl)-5-methyl-1,3,4-oxadiazole-2-carboxamide **31**. This was treated with hydroxylamine followed by dialkyl acetylenedicarboxylate to give methyl-2-[2-(5-methyl-1,3,4-oxadiazole-2-carboxamido)propan-2-yl]-1,6-dihydro-5-hydroxy-6-oxo-pyrimidine-4-carboxylate **32**. The reaction of intermediate **32** with *p*-fluoro benzylamine gave **33**. Methylation of **33** afforded Raltegravir **1**. The inventor disclosed that the Raltegravir obtained from this novel process has purity above 99.5% with an overall yield ranging from 55 to 58%.

Failure of Raltegravir-based treatment regimens to fully suppress HIV replication due to multiple viral amino acid mutations that confer resistance to Raltegravir **1** necessitated a search for improved anti-HIV integrase therapy [38].

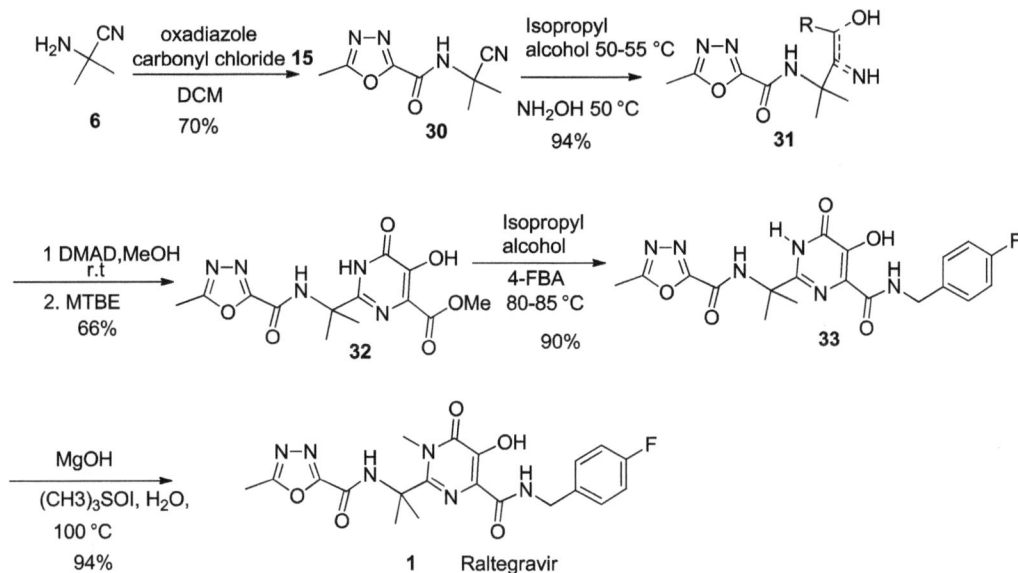

Scheme 5. Synthetic route for Raltegravir [37].

ELVITEGRAVIR

Background

A license agreement between Japan Tobacco and Gilead Sciences led to the clinical development of Elvitegravir **2** (EVG) [39, 40]. Elvitegravir **2** has the chemical name: 6-(3-chloro-2-fluoro-benzyl)-1-[(S)-1-hydroxy-methyl-2-methyl-propyl]-7-methoxy-4-oxo-1, 4-dihydro-quinoline-3-carboxylic acid. As compared to Raltegravir, the development of Elvitegravir is a major advancement in HIV treatment since it has a once-daily dosage however, its major drawback is its extensive cross resistance with Raltegravir [41].

Synthesis of Elvitegravir

Motomura *et al.* [40] first reported the synthesis of the novel integrase inhibitor JTK-303 (GS 9137), also known as Elvitegravir **2**, in 2006. The author described the modification of a quinolone antibiotic to produce JTK-303 (GS 9137) which blocks strand transfer by the viral enzyme. It shares the core structure of quinolone antibiotics and was shown to exhibit an IC_{50} of 7.2 nM in the strand transfer assay, and an EC_{50} of 0.9 nM in an acute HIV-1 infection assay.

The synthetic routes of Elvitegravir **2** described in Scheme (**6**), is based on a medicinal research paper on novel HIV–integrase inhibitor [40]. The synthesis starts from 2,4-difluorobenzoic acid **34** *via* iodination, acylation and condensation reactions to give ethyl 2-(2,4-difluoro-5-iodobenzoyl)-3-dimethylaminoacrylate **37**. The latter was then subjected to an addition-elimination reaction with (*S*)-valinol to give enamine **38** which was subsequently cyclized to quinolone **39**. **39** underwent hydroxyl protection with *tert*-butyldimethylsilyl chloride to afford carbonate **40a** which under the condition of Negishi coupling with 3-chloro-2-fluorobenzyl zinc bromide **42** in the presence of an organopalladium catalyst afforded quinolone ester **43a**. Subsequent one-pot synthesis of **43a** *via* alkaline deprotection afforded intermediate **44**. Methylation of the latter with sodium methoxide gave Elvitegravir **2** with an overall yield of 41%.

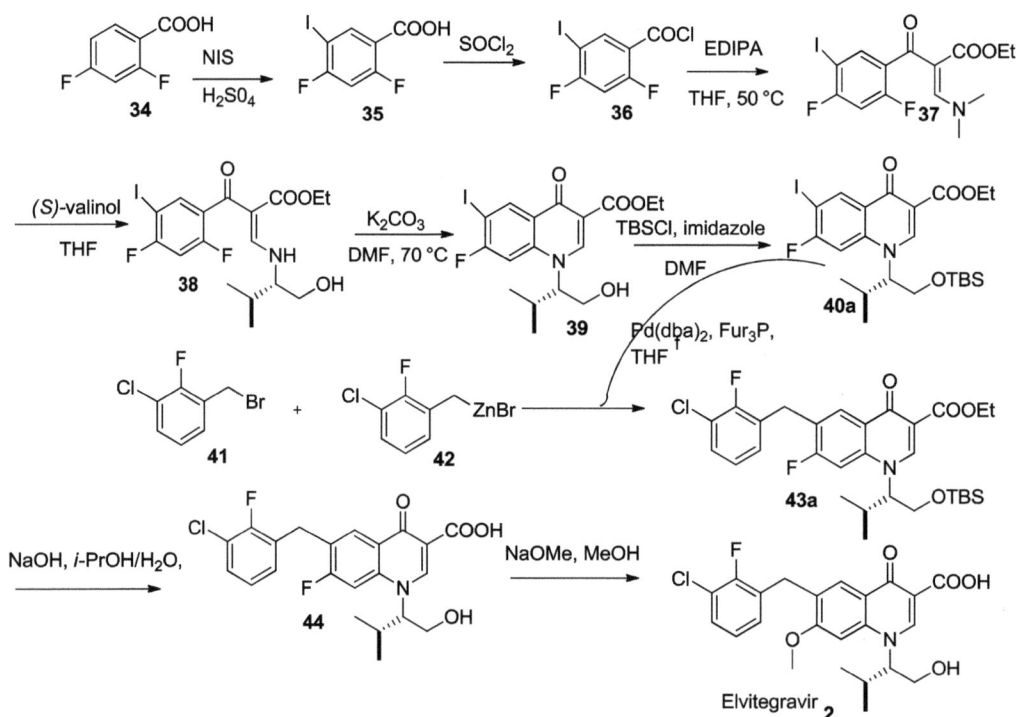

Scheme 6. Synthetic route of Elvitegravir [40].

The patent (Scheme **7**) by Japan Tobacco [39] disclosed two analogue synthetic routes to Elvitegravir **2**. These both rely on the use of 2,4-difluorobenzoic acid and share the same procedure with the previous medicinal synthetic route (Scheme **6**) except for the use of methylchloroformate to protect the hydroxyl group of **39** to give **40b** (Scheme **7**).

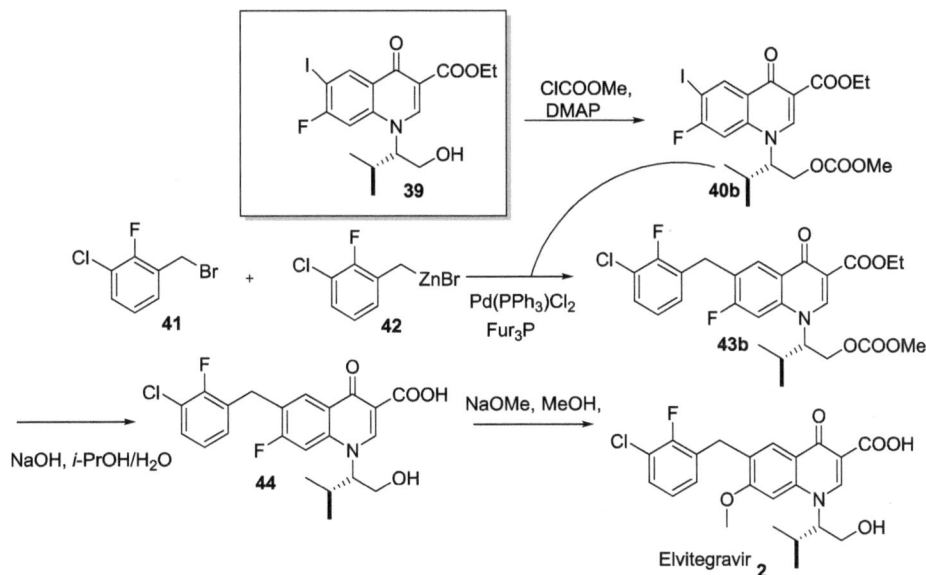

Scheme 7. Synthetic route of Elvitegravir [39].

Negishi coupling of **40b** with 3-chloro-2-fluorobenzyl zinc bromide **42** gave quinolone ester **43b**. Subsequent one-pot synthesis of **44** including deprotection, hydrolysis and methylation gave a crystalline form of Elvitegravir **2** with superior physical and chemical stability compared to other physical forms of the compound.

However, the said processes are tedious, lengthy and the penultimate intermediate **44**, a major impurity in the process, affected the purity of the final compound. In addition, an expensive compound, 2-fluoro-3-chlorobenzylbromide **41**, is used as a starting material for the synthesis of **2** thus there is a need for new cost effective synthetic methods of producing Elvitegravir. These methods should be easy to implement and have the ability to increase the yield and purity of the final compound as well as eliminate the use of toxic or costly reagents.

A process patent procedure [42] (Scheme **8**) on the other hand, begins with the commercially available 2,4-dimethoxybenzoic acid **45** which was converted into methyl ester **47** in three steps. The reaction of **47** with 3-chloro-2-fluorobenzylzinc bromide **42** gave the ester **48**, which was transformed to the ketoester **51** in the subsequent steps. The reaction of ketoester **51** with DMF-dimethylacetal afforded the benzoacrylate **52** which further reacted with (*S*)-(+)-valinol to give the enamine **53**. Cyclization of the enamine **53** afforded the quinolinone **55**. The hydroxyl group of **53** was protected with a reaction with *tert*-butyldimethylsilyl chloride and the resulting compound **54** was subsequently cyclised to the protected quinolone derivative **55**. Hydrolysis of the ethyl ester **55** as well as removal of the protecting TBDMS group afforded Elvitegravir **2**. The major disadvantage of this process is the early introduction of the most expensive reagent (2-fluoro-3-chlorobenzyl bromide).

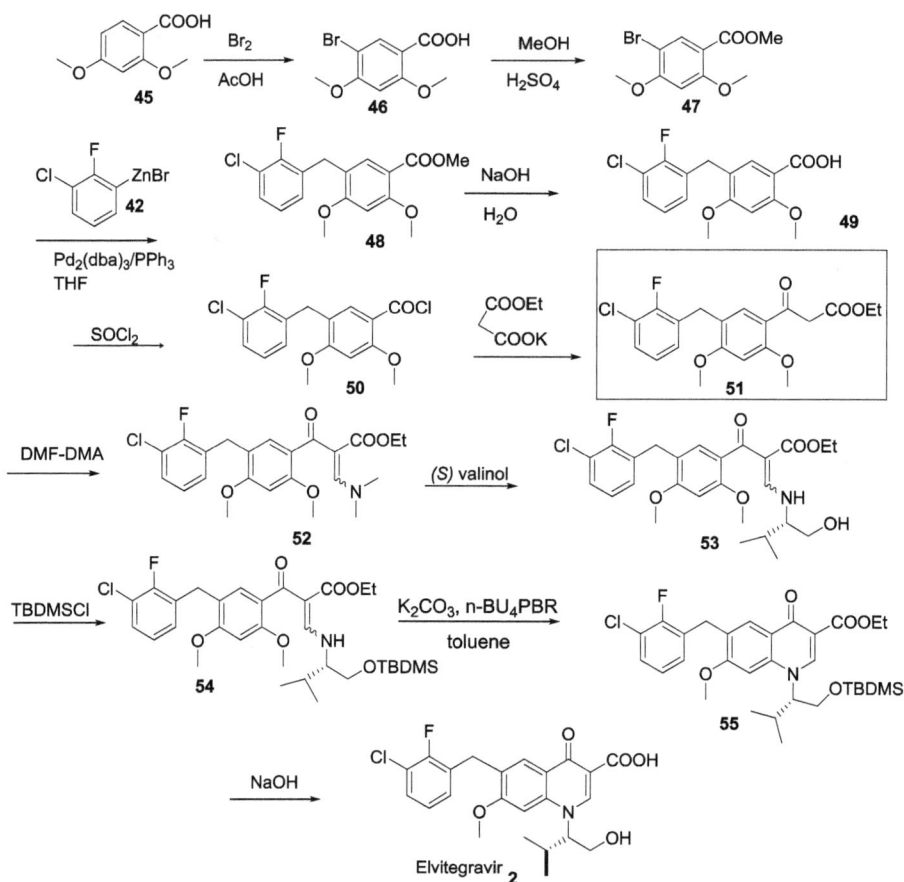

Scheme 8. Synthetic route of Elvitegravir.

Also, a recently published process patent from Gilead Sciences (Scheme **10**) [43] disclosed a method of preparing Elvitegravir **2** on kilogram scale using a similar synthetic protocol described in Scheme **9** but differs in the method of preparing the key intermediate **51**. Commercial 2,4-dimethoxy-5-bromobenzoic acid **56** was converted to magnesium salt when treated with butylethylmagnesium. Subsequent lithiation of the magnesium salt with *n*-butyllithium at -20 °C afforded the aryl lithium species. The aryl lithium species was then reacted with the 2-fluoro-3-chloro benzaldehyde **57** to give the hydroxyl acid **58**. Reduction of the hydroxyl group with triethylsilane in TFA afforded benzoic acid **59**. This acid was then reacted with carbonyldiimidazole to give the imidazole functional derivative **60** which subsequently reacted with potassium ethyl malonate to give ketoester **51** after workup. The condensation with DMF–DMA converted ketoester **51** to the benzoacrylate **61** which was immediately subjected to an addition–elimination reaction involving (*S*)-valinol in toluene at ambient temperature to give enamine **62**. Warming the resulting intermediate **62** in the presence of *N,O*-bistrimethylsilyl acetamide (BSA) and potassium chloride in DMF afforded the ring-closed quinolone **63**. Saponification of the ester **63** was achieved with potassium hydroxide in aqueous isopropanol followed by acidification and crystallization to afford Elvitegravir **2**. Despite both routes employing the same key fragments, the Gilead process route is superior in the sense that it is more scalable and involves fewer reaction steps.

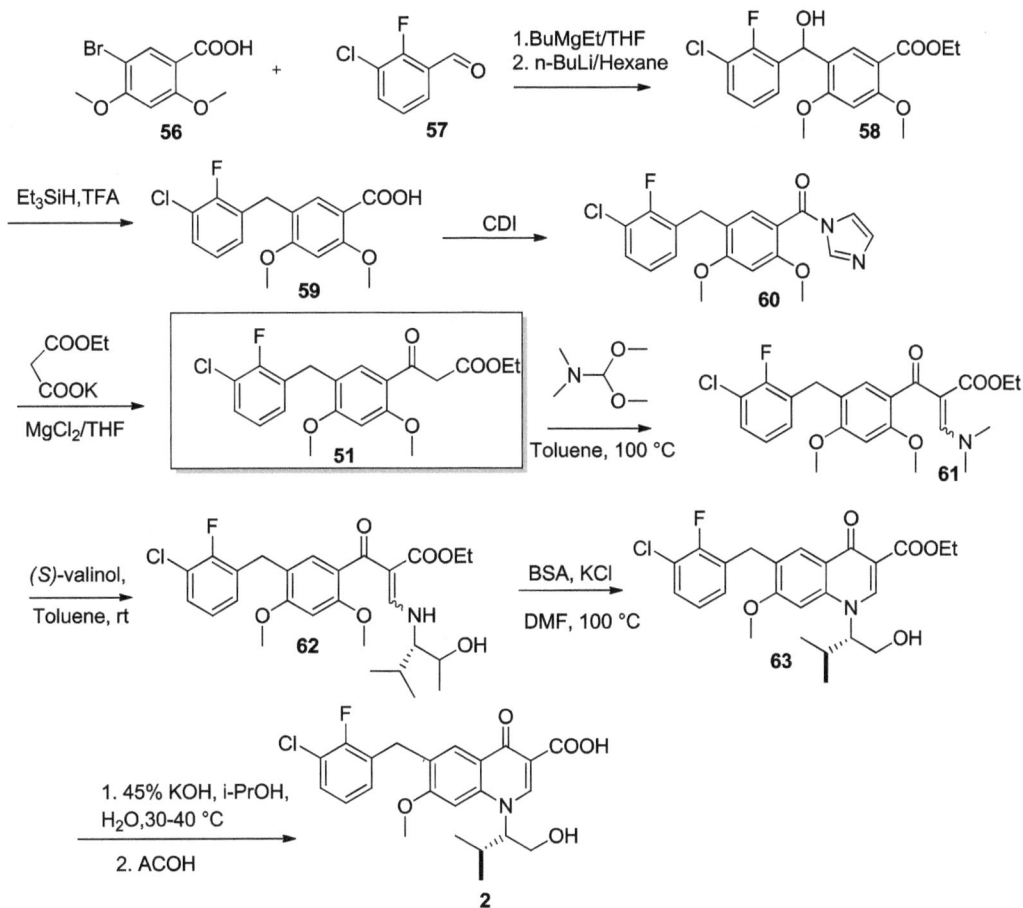

Scheme 9. Synthetic route of Elvitegravir [43].

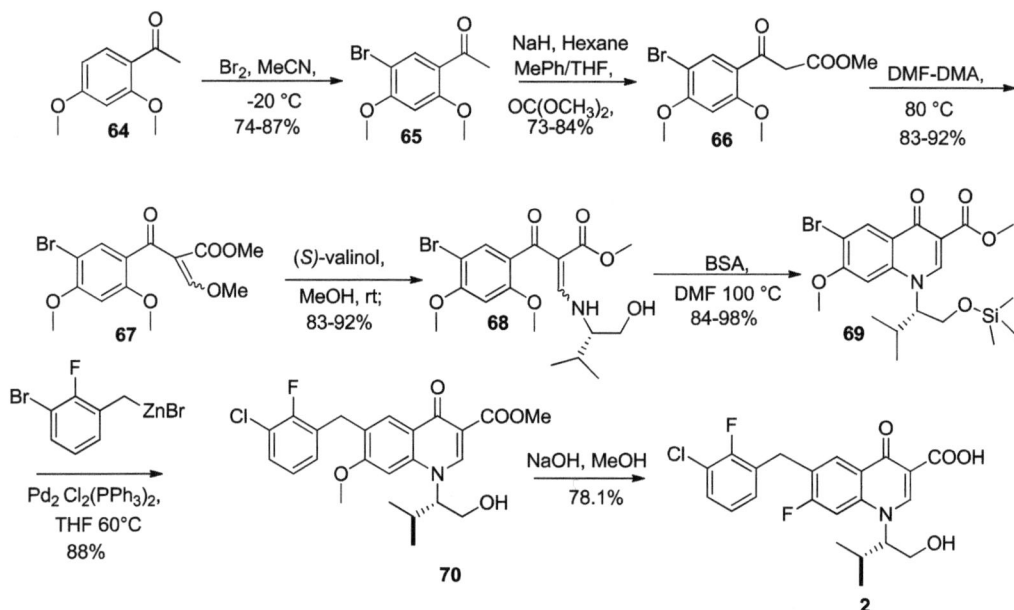

Scheme 10. Synthetic route of Elvitegravir [44].

Another improved process for the synthesis of Elvitegravir was patented [44](Scheme **10**) and begins with commercially available 2,4-dimethoxy-acetophenone **64**, which was selectively halogenated at the position 5 to give 5-bromo acetophenone **65**. Condensation of **65** with dimethyl carbonates provided benzoylacetate **66**. Treatment of **66** with *N,N*-dimethylformamide dimethyl acetal followed by (*S*)-valinol gave the corresponding intermediate benzoyl acrylate **68**. Aromatic nucleophilic substitution of the 2-methoxy group with 2.2-5.0 equivalents of *N,O*-bis(trimethylsilyl)-acetamide which also protected the OH group as the trimethylsilyl derivative gave 1,4-dihydroquinolin-4-oxo derivatives **69**. Negishi coupling of **69** with 2-fluoro-3-chlorobenzylzinc bromide followed by hydrolysis provided Elvitegravir **2** in 29.3% yield from a total of seven reaction steps.

The use of 2.2-5.0 equivalents of *N,O*-bis(trimethylsilyl)-acetamide offered an improvement to the original procedure reported by Satoh *et al.* [39] which utilized an expensive *tert*-butyldimethylsilyl chloride. In addition, the expensive chloro-2-fluorobenzyl group was introduced in the final stage of the synthesis thus making this route cost effective.

Raltegravir **1** and Elvitegravir **2** have relatively low genetic barriers to resistance and they share a high degree of cross-resistance which led to the development of the second-generation integrase drugs [45].

DOLUTEGRAVIR

Background

Dolutegravir (DTG) **3** (also known as S/GSK 13495672), a second-generation integrase inhibitor, was developed by Glaxo Smith Kline and its Japanese partner, Shionogi for the treatment of HIV infection. It was FDA approved in August 2013. DTG has potential advantages in comparison to first-generation INSTI's, including unboosted daily dosing, limited cross resistance with Raltegravir **1** and Elvitegravir **2** as well as a high genetic barrier to resistance [13]. DTG has also been recommended as a preferred first-line antiretroviral drug therapy.

Synthesis of Dolutegravir

Several publications and patents [46, 47] including process patents describing preparation of the key fragments and full synthesis of Dolutegravir have been published. The first description of the synthesis of Dolutegravir (Scheme **11**) was described in a patent WO 2006/16764 in 16 steps. An alternative synthesis (Scheme **12**) was described in WO 2010/068253 (12 steps); using a novel pyrone and a pyridone derivatives.

However, the above production methods of Dolutegravir are not satisfactory for the industrial manufacturing process because of the followings: 1). long reaction process of about 16 or 11 steps (Schemes **11** and **12** respectively), 2). low yield, 3). the use of highly toxic selenium compounds and 4). the use expensive palladium catalyst [48]. The scalable process routes that have been disclosed within patent and published literatures for the synthesis of Dolutegravir **3** starting from available commercial materials are described below.

Yukihito *et al.* [49] (Scheme **13**) reported the process of preparation of dolutegravir starting from ethyl 3-oxobutanoate **95**. Firstly, enaminone **96** was obtained *via* reaction with Vilsmeier reagent (DMF acetal). This was then followed by the initial nucleophilic attack at dimethylamino methylene **96** by acid chloride **97** resulting in deprotonation of **96** with LiHMDS in THF at -78 °C and subsequent acidification with HCl to effect cyclisation with the elimination of dimethylamine to give the pyrone ester **98** in 43% yield. The reaction of the pyrone ester **98** with primary amine **99** afforded the pyridone derivative **100** in excellent yield (94%). Bromination of this intermediate gave the product **101** which was subsequently acidified with formic acid and sulphuric acid to give the amino acetaldehyde dimethyl acetal **102**. The aldehyde **104** underwent condensation with amino alcohol **103** to give tricyclic compound **104**. Alkaline hydrolysis of bromide from **104** followed by protection and coupling with amine

80 in the presence of HATU and NMO in DMF provided the title compound dolutegravir **3** in 73% yield.

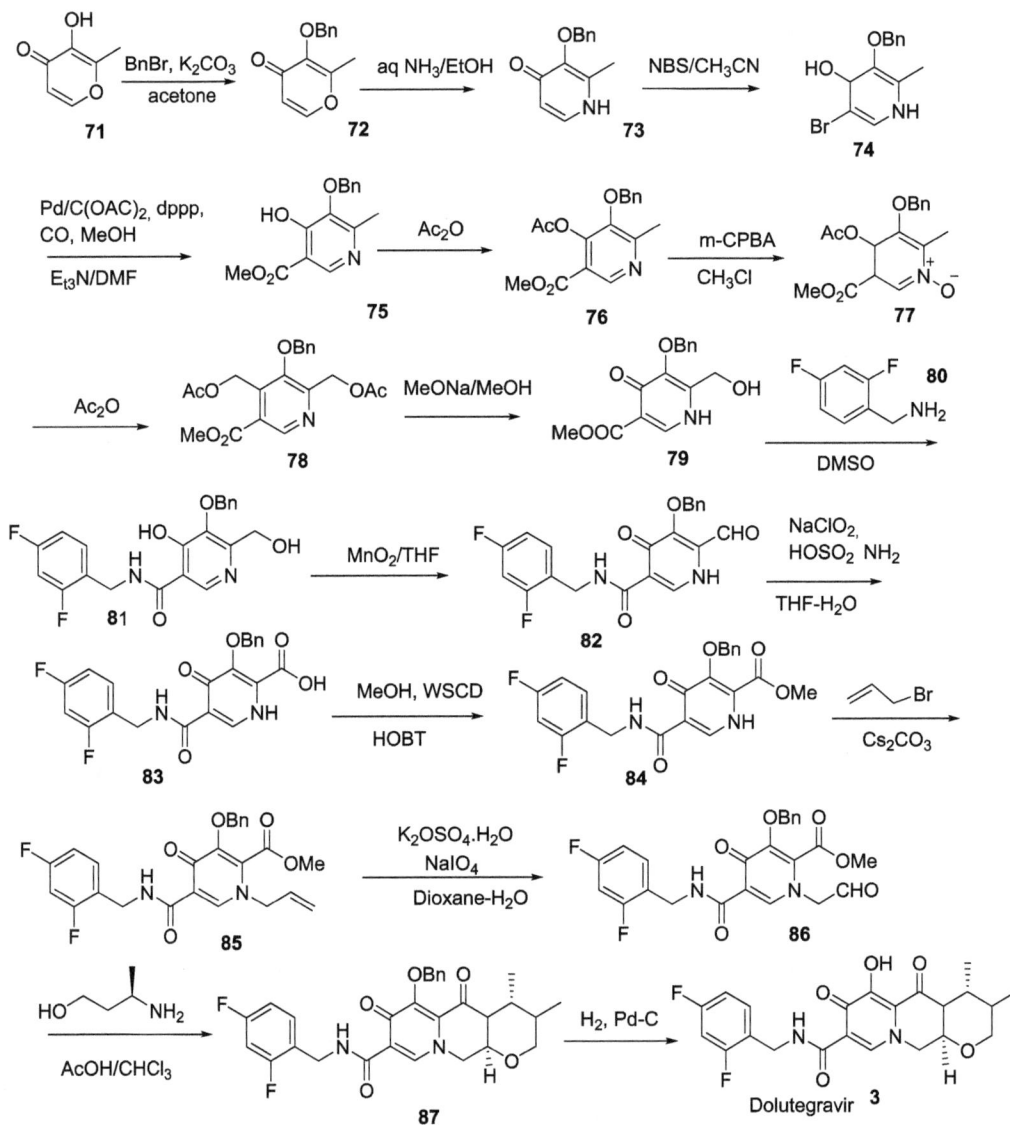

Scheme 11. Synthesis of Dolutegravir.

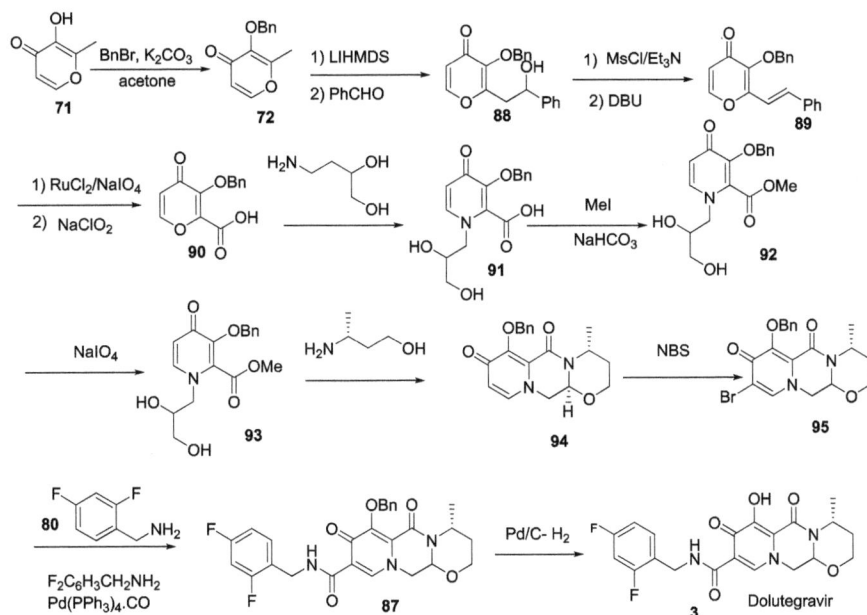

Scheme 12. Synthesis of Dolutegravir.

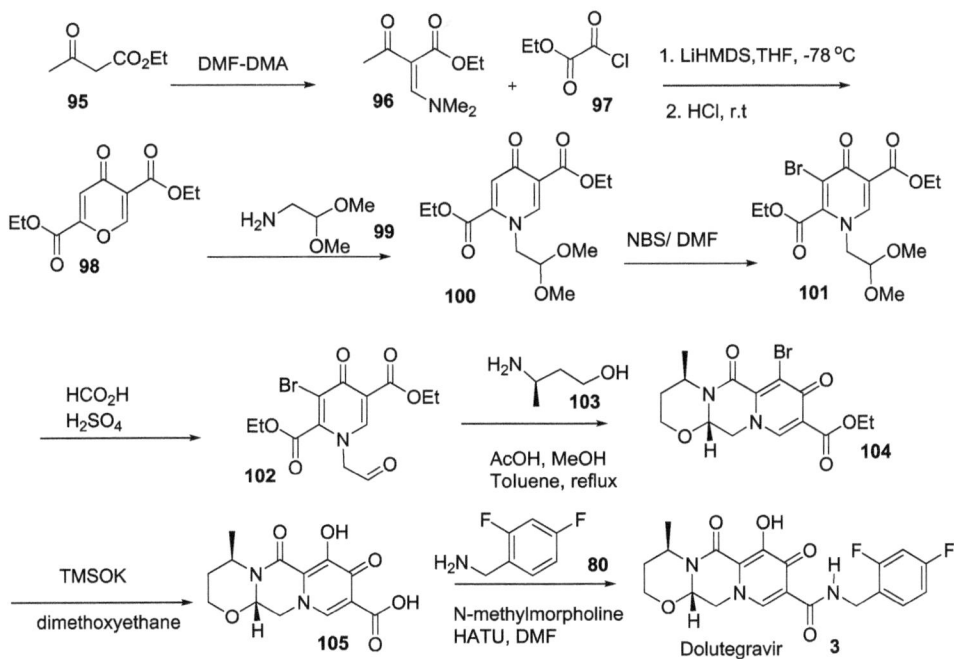

Scheme 13. Synthesis of dolutegravir [49].

Wang *et al.* [50] disclosed a very different approach to access Dolutegravir **3** as shown in Scheme **14** starting from methyl-4-(methoxy)-3-oxobutanoate **106**. Treatment of **106** with 1,1-dimethoxy *N,N*-dimethylmethanamine gave the enaminone **107** from which subsequent treatment with **99** afforded intermediate **108**. Condensation of **108** with dimethyl oxalate in the presence of lithium methanolate at 40 °C gave the dimethylester **110**. Addition of LiOH at 5 °C regioselectively saponified dimethylester **110** to **111**. Acidic cleavage of the ketal with MsOH/AcOH in acetonitrile gave the free aldehyde **112** and condensation with **103** gave the tricyclic acid **113**. CDI-mediated coupling of **113** with **80** afforded 7-*O*-protected Dolutegravir **3**. Cleavage of the methyl ether with MgBr$_2$ in acetonitrile at 50 °C gave Dolutegravir **3**.

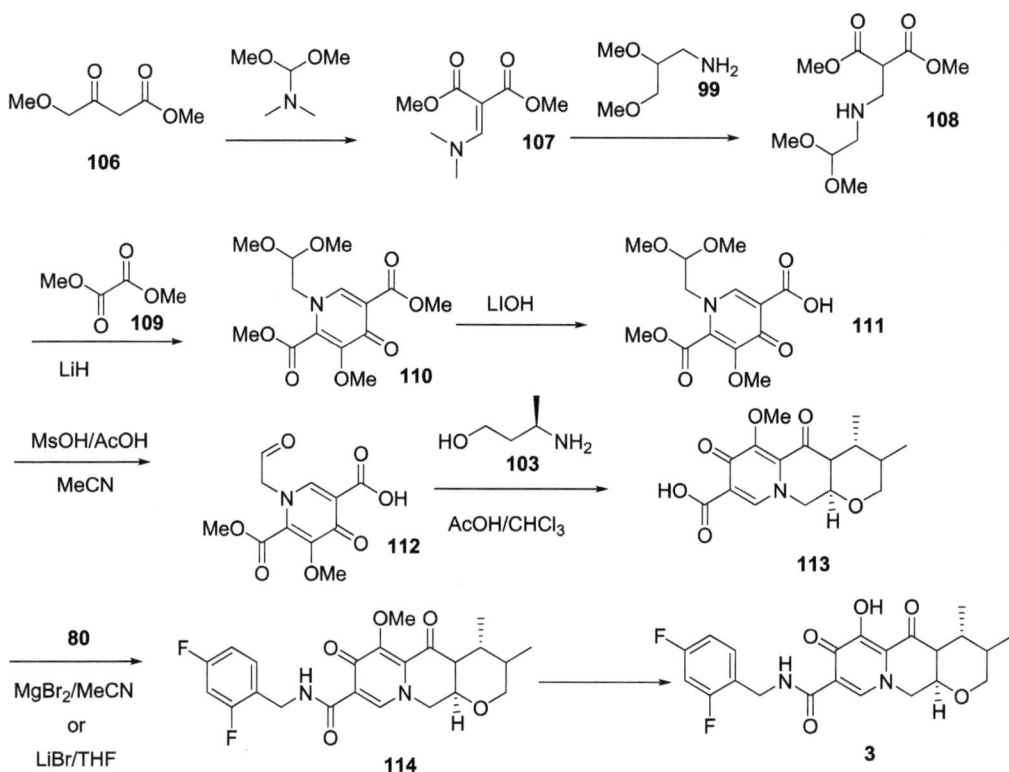

Scheme 14. Synthesis of Dolutegravir [50].

Sankareswaran *et al.* [51] described a four-stage manufacturing route for the preparation of Dolutegravir sodium (Scheme **16**) which appears to be high yielding and a scalable process. The key improvements in their process include the development of mild workup procedure by selective derivatization of a process impurity using *tert*-butyldimethylsilyl chloride. The critical isomeric impurity was identified and eliminated *via* establishment of proper control strategy and the optimization of metal-based hydrogenation-free *O*-debenzylation was also carried out. The synthesis (Scheme **15**) begins with a key intermediate **118** in whose synthetic route was reported in a patent by Sumino *et al.* (Scheme **16**) [48].

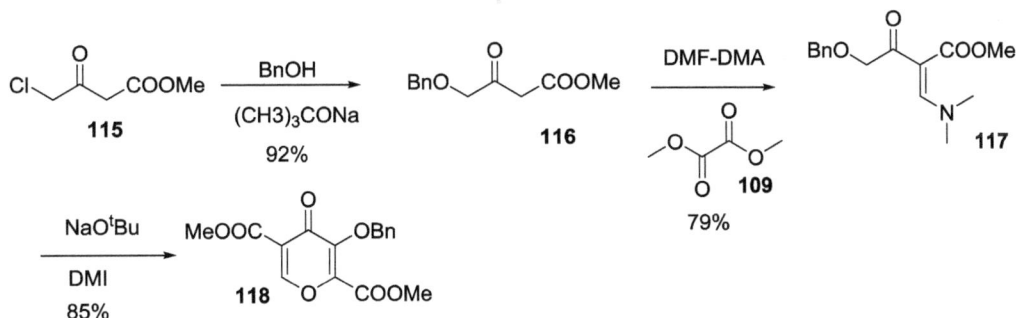

Scheme 15. Synthesis of Dolutegravir intermediate **118** [48].

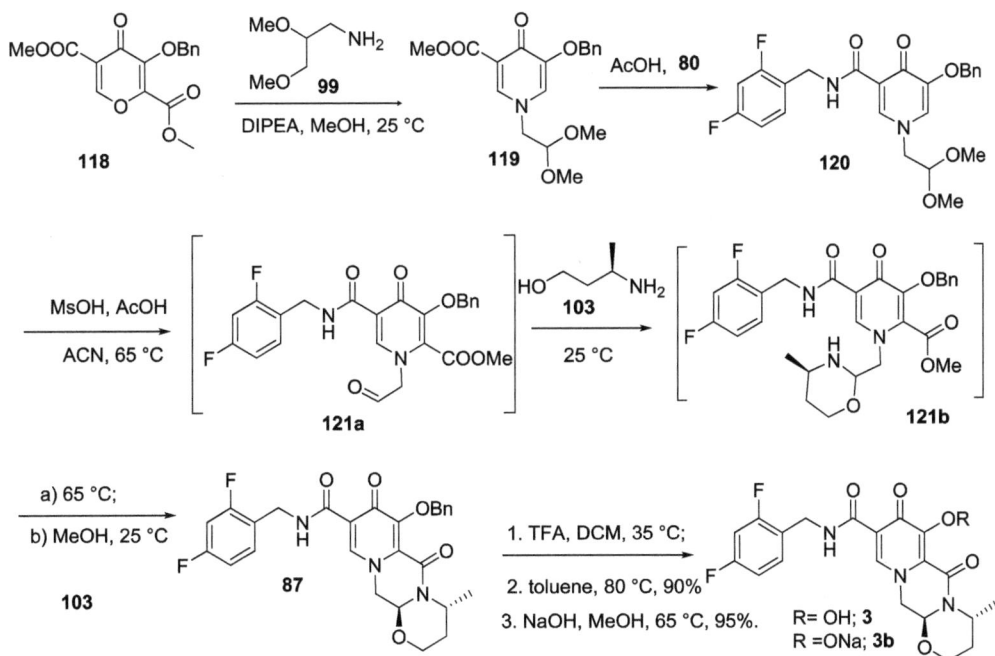

Scheme 16. Synthesis of dolutegravir [51].

The synthesis of **118** begins with deprotonation of benzyl alcohol with sodium *tert*-pentoxide. The resulting phenyl methoxide intermediate then undergoes nucleophilic substitution with the chlorine of methyl 4-chloroacetoacetate **115** to give compound **116** in 92% yield. Condensation reaction of **116** with dimethyl oxalate in the presence of DMF-DMA afforded dimethyl-3-(benzyloxy)-4-oxo-4-*H*-pyran-2,5-dicarboxylate **118** in 85% yield.

Sankareswaran *et al.* [51] reported one of the most efficient, economical and process friendly routes by using commercially available dimethyl-3-(benzyloxy)-4-oxo-4-*H*-pyran-2,5-dicarb-oxylate **118** to access dolutegravir **3** (Scheme **16**). Reaction of **118** with 2,2-dimethoxyethanamine **99** opened the pyran ring **118** which later cyclized back to give the pyridine analogue **119** as an oil. This was then followed by regioselective reaction of **119** with 2,4 diflourobenzylamine **80** in the presence of acetic acid to give amidoester **120**. Acidic cleavage of the dimethyl ketal followed by reaction with *3R* aminobutanol in the presence of acid gave chiral hemiaminal **121b** which underwent diastereoselective cyclization to form benzyl protected dolutegravir intermediate **87**. Simultaneous debenzylation of **87** followed by salification with aqueous sodium hydroxide afforded dolutegravir sodium **3b**.

BICTEGRAVIR

Background

Bictegravir [BIC (GS-9883) **4**, is the most recently approved INST (Feb 7, 2018) that is used in combination with tenofovir alafenamide (TAF) and emtricitabine (FTC) as a once-daily single tablet regimen for the treatment of HIV/AIDS infection [52]. It has low to no cytotoxicity with an improved pharmacokinetics and *in vitro* resistance profile relative to compounds **1-3** against patient-derived isolates resistant to INSTIs. Combination of Bictegravir with approved antiretroviral drugs such as nucleoside reverse transcriptase inhibitors NRTIs (TAF and FTC) or with darunavir (DRV), a protease inhibitor (PI) was highly synergistic. Breakthrough resistance studies indicate that **4** has a higher barrier to *in vitro* resistance emergence compared with Raltegravir **1** or Elvitegravir **2** and is similar to Dolutegravir **3**.

Synthesis of Bictegravir

The discovery synthesis of Bictegravir BIC **4** was reported in a patent US2014/0221356 A1 [53]. The discovery synthesis of Bictegravir paralleled the discovery route of Dolutegravir (Scheme **13**) from **106** through **107** to provide **122**, The synthesis of **4** starts with the preparation of a key intermediate 1-(2,2-dimethoxy-ethyl)-5-methoxy-6-(methoxy-carbonyl)-4-oxo-1,4-dihydro-pyridine-3-carboxylic acid **122** invented by Wang *et al.* which was patented in WO2011/119566A1 [50]. Coupling of compound **122** with 2,4 diflourobenzylamine **80** and DIPEA in the presence of HATU gave **123**. The resulting **123** was converted to **124** in the presence of methanesuphonic acid. Heating of **124** with 3-aminocyclopentanol followed by methyl deprotection with magnesium bromide afforded Bictegravir **4** as a racemic mixture in eight steps, however, the product yield was not disclosed in this patent.

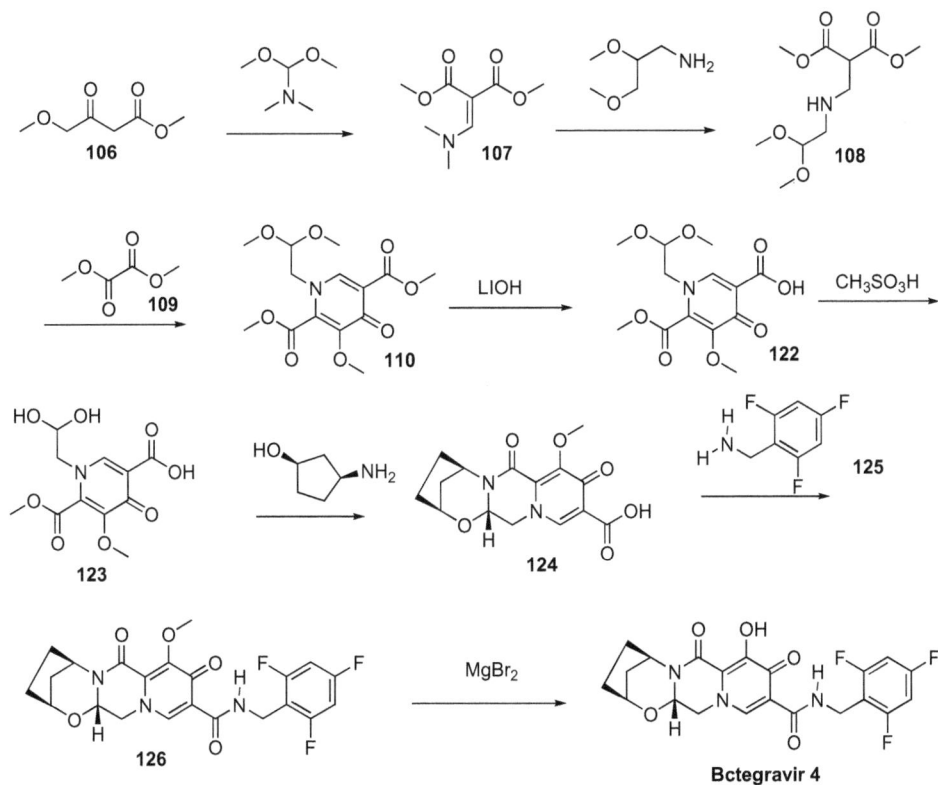

Scheme 17. Synthesis of Bictegravir [53].

Batch synthesis, as has been illustrated in the above syntheses, still takes up a very large part of production in the pharmaceutical, fine chemicals and food industry. However, there is a need for enabling technology which is greener and cost effective.

ORGANIC SYNTHESIS IN THE PHARMA INDUSTRY

Background

For centuries, chemical reactions have been carried out in the batch mode of processing where an increase in output is directly proportional to the size of the reaction vessels. This mode of production is commonly used in low volume throughput industries (fine chemical and specialty chemicals) and may not be convenient for certain type of productions *i.e.* the high volume industries *e.g.* the petroleum industry, which relies on continuous mode of processing. There are two general types of conventional reactors; batch and continuous flow reactors. The batch reactor is usually made of stainless steel or glass lined steel vessel with a mixer, cooling and heating jackets [54]. The common problems encountered in these reactors are poor mass and heat transfer due to inadequate mixing which in turn can cause hot spots and high concentration of reactants in some parts of the vessel. The continuous flow reactor on the other hand is categorized into fixed bed reactors and plug flow reactors where the concentration of components in the reaction remains essentially constant after proper mixing. Both types of conventional processing have disadvantages and advantages. It is definitely unsurprising that each of these modes of processing have their own defined niche in the chemical production industry.

Even with the available new technologies *i.e.* down scaled continuous flow, processing that could revolutionize processing in the fine chemical industry, a change from the traditional batch processing to flow processing is still at a snail pace. A survey carried out to determine the status of the implementation of continuous processing among the roundtable member organizations, found that the challenges affecting the implementation included; 1). High level of uncertainty as to whether the process will deliver to justify its implementation, 2). The various stages involved in drug development do not favor changes in method of processing, 3). Lack of need to invest in new technology yet the existing one provides substantial production capacity, 4). Lack of experienced personnel to implement the technology and troubleshoot in case problems are encountered and lastly the lack of equipment for scaling processes to industrial capacity [55].

The regulatory bodies as Plumb [56] puts it, also have to recognize the role of continuous processing more so since the industry depends on certain manufacturing practices coupled with manufacturing & product licenses which take relatively a long period to acquire. It is worth mentioning that the FDA has now recently shown an interest in encouraging and accepting the use of newer technologies and safer manufacturing practices in the pharmaceutical industry [57]. This has led to a snowballed eagerness from the pharma industry players towards continuous flow processing [22]. This is also evident from the growing number of continuous flow synthesis processes for APIs and precursors being developed and patented [58]. This change in mind-set is hugely attributed to the support from the FDA.

CONTINUOUS FLOW PROCESSING AND THE PHARMA INDUSTRY

Continuous flow processing involves carrying out of chemical transformations in a tubular structure with dimensions ranging between microliter and millilitre scale. This is becoming a common technique for organic syntheses especially in the research laboratories. At this level, many a research group have demonstrated the numerous advantages it brings forth to a variety of chemical syntheses. Some advantages that have been showcased in literature [20, 59, 60] include shorter reaction times, excellent yields and selectivity, high throughput, enhanced safety, improved mass & heat transfers in addition to rapid parameter screening and easy reaction scale up to mention but a few. These advantages are attributed to the large surface area to volume ratio, small reactor dimensions and the ability to enable telescoping of reaction steps. Most of these have been exploited in API synthesis and drug development [20, 61 - 63]. In this section, we focus on demystifying the benefits of HIV drugs and API synthesis in continuous flow systems. Examples of some of the molecules discussed are shown in Fig. (3) below.

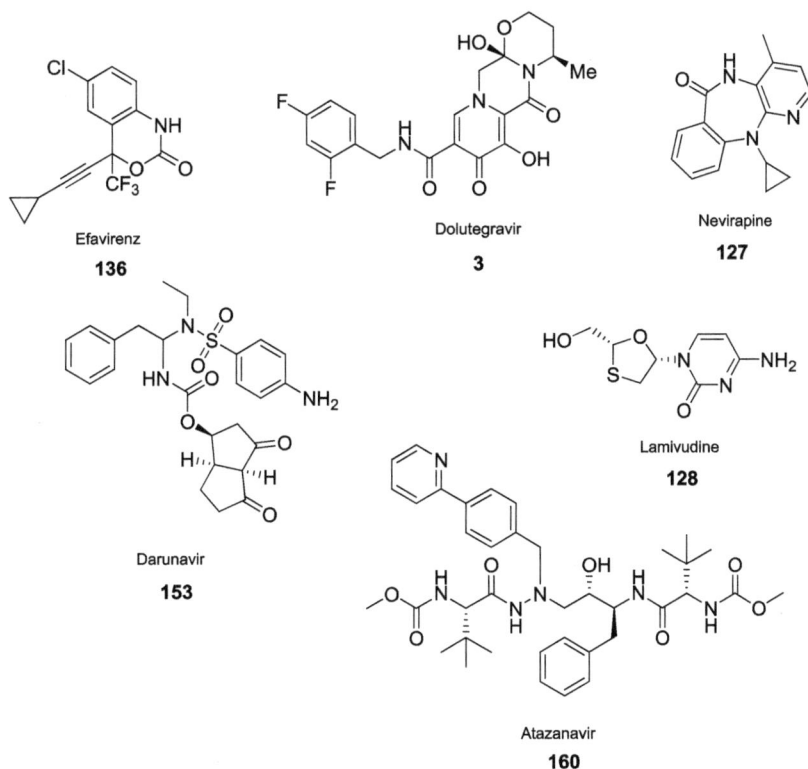

Fig. (3). Continuous flow synthesized potent molecules used in the treatment of HIV.

APPLICATION OF CONTINUOUS FLOW PROCESSING IN HIV/AIDS DRUGS AND APIS SYNTHESIS

CONTINUOUS FLOW SYNTHESIS OF NEVIRAPINE PRECURSOR

Nevirapine **127**, also called Viramune, is a non-nucleosidic reverse transcriptase inhibitor (NNRTI) used in antiretroviral therapy. In 1996, it was approved by the Food and Drug Administration for the treatment of HIV [64]. Nevirapine, in combination with Lamuvidine (3TC) **128** and Azidothymidine (AZT) or Tenofovir (TDF), is one of the preferred first-line combination drug therapies recommended by the World Health Organisation. With the unending HIV scourge, it is paramount to improve the synthesis of these drugs either by using better chemistries or cheaper and readily available raw materials, which culminate into lower process and production costs. Thus far, most existing syntheses of Nevirapine are performed in batch reactors of which these methods are usually marred with long reaction times and selectivity issues. In a bid to reduce Nevirapine production costs, Mcquade *et al.* have explored the continuous flow synthesis of 2-bromo-4-methylnicotinonitrile **129**, a nicotinonitrile precursor to Nevirapine **127** [19]. The precursor **129** was obtained in 69% yield after a 45 minute batch cyclization of crude enamine **130** that was synthesised from a three-step telescoped synthesis consisting of acetone **131** and malononitrile **132** as starting substrates (Fig. **4**). The synthesis of Isopropylidenemalononitrile **133**, and Knoevenagel condensation steps were elegantly telescoped by introducing a packed bed of 3 Å molecular sieves to absorb water from the first step before the addition of DMF-DMA. It was also illustrated that reactant concentration affected the stability of the Al_2O_3 column. A Knoevenagel concentration of 0.5 M and an Al_2O_3 column heated at 95 °C was found to provide long-term column stability. In a total residence time of 5.75 minutes, the crude enamine **130** was obtained.

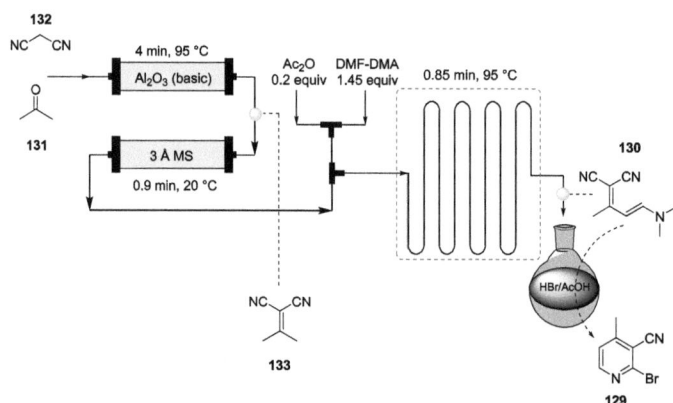

Fig. (4). Continuous flow synthesis of an intermediate towards Nevirapine.

This investigation is a step towards an easy and rapid continuous flow synthesis of Nevirapine precursor. 0.37 g of Al_2O_3 and 0.28 g of molecular sieves was needed to attain 1 g of product **129** in comparison to the batch synthesis, which required 0.98 g of catalyst to attain the same amount product.

CONTINUOUS FLOW SYNTHESIS OF DOLUTEGRAVIR

Jamison *et al*. have reported a 7-step flow synthesis of Dolutegravir **3**, a second generation HIV integrase strand transfer inhibitor used for the treatment of HIV-1 infections [23]. This was adapted from a reported GlaxoSmithKline process chemistry batch route for Cabotegravir. The flow synthesis was achieved through a one by one reaction step optimisation approach prior to telescoping of steps. Solvent screening was carried out in batch for reaction steps that were to be telescoped in flow. The investigation of the flow synthesis of Dolutegravir **3** was started from the condensation of methyl-4-methoxyacetoacetate **108** with **99**. In a residence time of 10 minutes, at 85 °C and 1.6 equivalents of DMF-DMA, full conversion of **108** to **99** was attained. This step and the synthesis of vinylogous amide **107**, were thereafter telescoped from which 95% of vinylogous amide was obtained in 8 minutes with a throughput of 43 gh^{-1}. An optimised pyridone flow synthesis of **110** was also successfully added thus creating a fully continuous three-step synthesis (Fig. **5**). In a total residence time of 74 minutes, a 54% isolated yield of **110** and a throughput of 3.4 gh^{-1} was obtained.

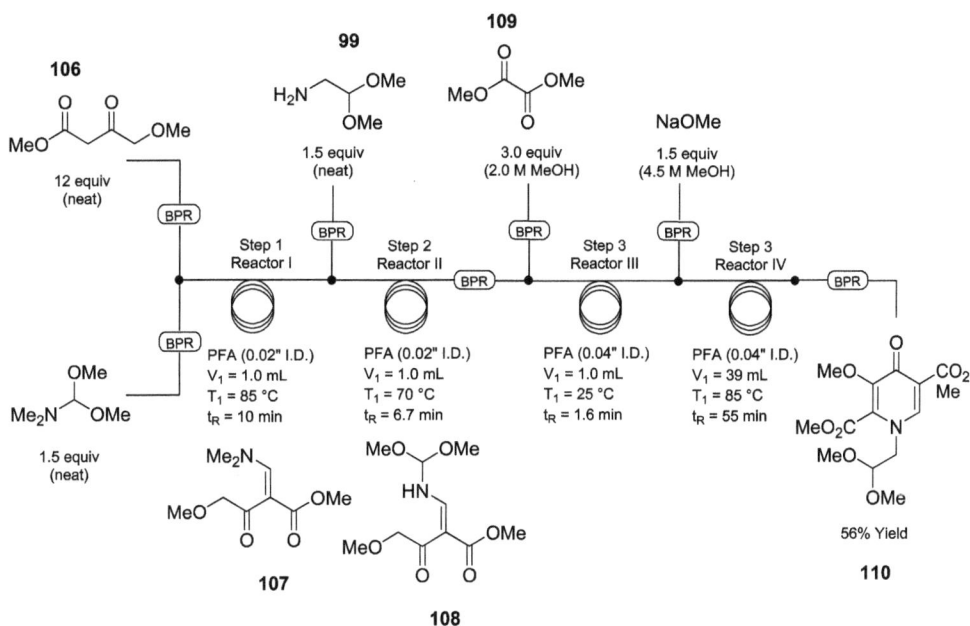

Fig. (5). A Three-step telescoped pyridone flow synthesis towards Dolutegravir.

Both base and acid promoted direct amidation of **110** were also investigated. It was found that the acid catalysed reaction took longer than the base catalysed amidation. On a 3 mmol scale, 5 equivalents of Acetic acid, a reaction temperature of 200 °C, 96% yield of amide **134** was obtained in 124 minutes (throughput of 3.5 gh⁻¹). In contrast, LiOMe or NaOMe in mixed solvent system of methanol and toluene shortened the reaction time to 35 minutes and gave 95% yield at 80 °C. Unfortunately, attempts to telescope this protocol with the previous steps were futile due to extensive clogging.

The workers hereafter embarked on optimising the continuous flow deprotection of acetal **134** and cyclization with (*R*)-3-aminobutan-1-ol **103** based on batch screening experiments. An initial attempt in flow, led to very low yield (5%, 5:1 dr) and formation of by-product **135**, a result of elimination of hemi-aminal ether functionality and deprotected pyridine in 24% yield. This was due to the one-step flow protocol used. The synthesis of **114** was thereafter successfully achieved by carrying out the synthesis in a two-step flow protocol. This change enabled the use of a stoichiometric amount of *p*-toulene sulfonic acid as opposed to the neat formic acid used in their initial attempt. Additionally, there was no elimination by-product **135** observed. **114** was furnished in a total residence time of 66 minutes at a reaction temperature of 100 °C, the deprotection of acetal **134** and cyclization with (*R*)-3-aminobutan-1-ol **103** was telescoped with the previous step *i.e.* acid catalysed direct amidation of **110**. In 290 minutes, compound **114** was obtained in 48% yield. A three step telescoped flow synthesis of **114** was successfully attained (Fig. **6**).

The workers concluded their investigation with a stand-alone flow synthesis of **3** starting from purified **114**. The batch screened conditions for the demethylation of **114**, where LiBr was identified as suitable demethylating reagent and temperatures higher than 120 °C were found to lead to by-product formation, were also used to streamline a continuous flow protocol showed in Fig. (**6**). An 89% yield of **3** was reported to have been obtained within a residence time of 31 minutes at 100 °C (Fig. **7**). Jamison and co-workers successfully translated seven batch reaction steps in the synthesis of Dolutegravir **3** to flow synthesis. In addition, short reaction times, good yield and selectivity; benefits of continuous flow processing, were showcased in the telescoped and stand-alone flow protocols developed. In the grand scale of things, this in turn will ultimately shorten the manufacture to market times as well as reduce the cost of production of Dolutegravir; therefore, providing more and easy access of the drug to infected persons.

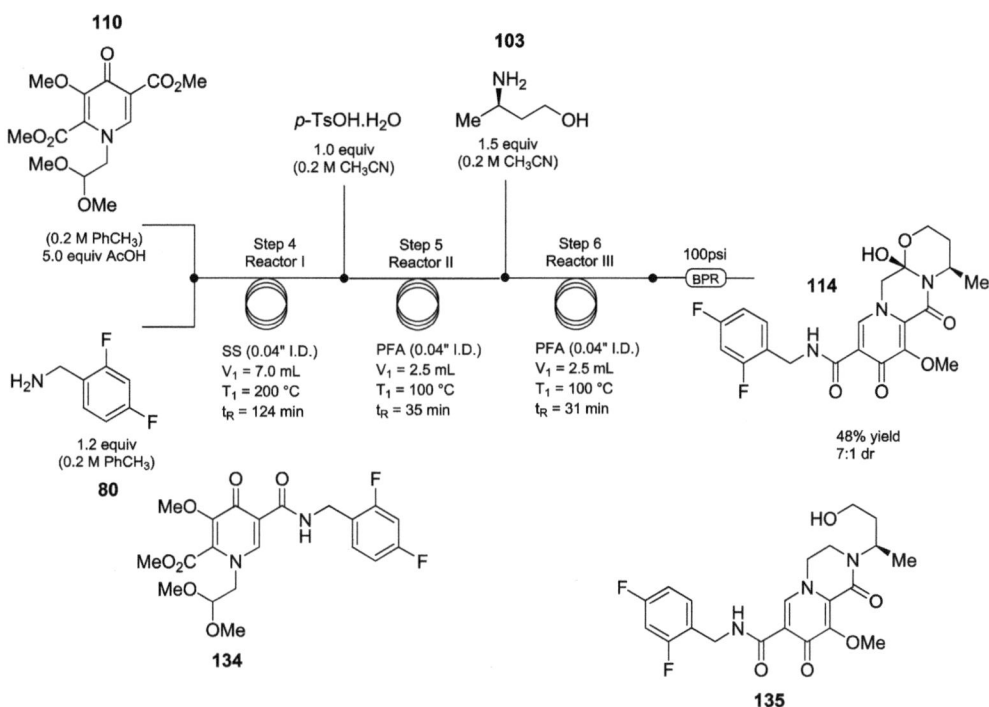

Fig. (6). Three-step telescoped flow synthesis of amide derivative.

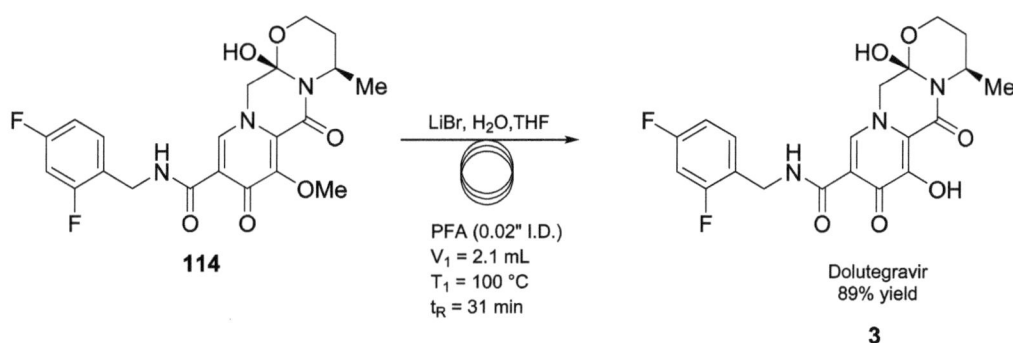

Fig. (7). Continuous flow demethylation in the synthesis of Dolutegravir.

CONTINUOUS FLOW SYNTHESIS OF EFAVIRENZ AND ITS INTERMEDIATES

Efavirenz **136** is an NNRTI used in combination therapy for first-line treatment of HIV [65]. There are only two major routes towards the synthesis of Efavirenz reported to date *i.e.* Merck and Lonza routes. The Merck route consists of five reaction steps starting from 4-chloroaniline whereas the Lonza route compromises of four steps starting from 1,4-dichlorobenze **137**. Chada *et al.* recently reported a continuous flow synthesis of an intermediate towards Efavirenz starting from *N*-Boc 4-chloroaniline **138** [25]. In this synthesis, *n*-butyllithium was used to facilitate the *ortho*-lithiation of *N*-Boc 4-chloroaniline **139**. Using a flexible flow reactor set up, they were able to determine the optimum reaction temperature, residence time and reagent concentration for the synthesis. Furthermore, a packed bed of anhydrous silica, which enabled in-line reaction quench, was effortlessly added to the microreactor system as shown in Fig. (**8**).

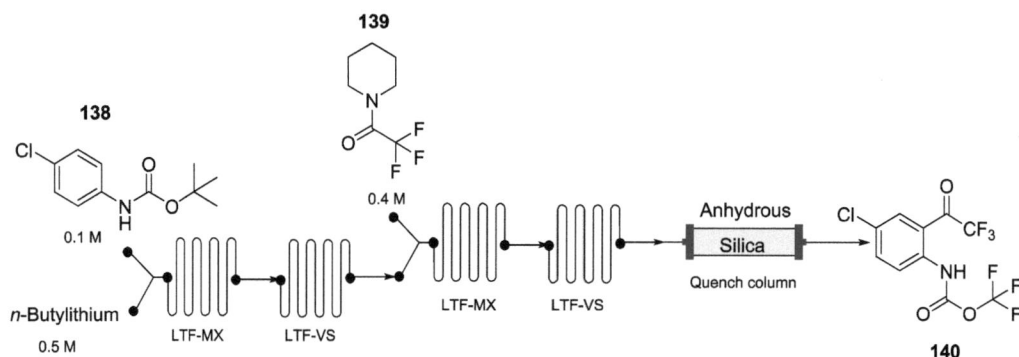

Fig. (8). Continuous flow *ortho*-lithiation of *N*-Boc 4-chloroaniline, an intermediate towards Efavirenz.

Accurate reaction parameter control was demonstrated in this synthesis moreover, the *ortho*-lithiation was successfully performed at temperatures high than the norm (-78 °C). Between -70 and -40 °C, a maximum conversion of 30% was recorded from a 0.5 M *n*-butyllithium, 0.1 M of *N*-Boc protected aniline **138** and 0.14 M piperidine trifluoroacetic acid **139** at a total flow rate of 0.13 mL/min and a residence time of 8.6 minutes. A decrease in *n*-BuLi concentration to 0.25 M had no effect on the conversion at the above-mentioned reaction conditions. On the other hand, increasing the concentration of trifluoroacylating agent **138** played a major role in improving the conversion of aniline **138** to intermediate **140**. Using 0.25 M *n*-BuLi, 0.1 M of **138** at -45 °C and a 0.2 M concentration of **138**, led to a 40% improvement in conversion of **138** to **140**. The flow synthesis of intermediate **140** *via* the *ortho*-lithiation of *N*-Boc protected chloroaniline **138** and trifluoroacylation using **139** provided a higher conversion at higher temperatures, lower equivalents of *n*-BuLi and in the absence of tetramethylethylenediame (TMEDA) than its batch synthesis (28% at -78 °C and 5 equivalents of *n*-BuLi). Additionally, the flow reactor system ensured process safety and rapid parameter optimisation with the use of small reagent volumes.

From prior literature, Seeberger and co-workers reported a continuous flow synthesis of Efavirenz following the Lonza route which involves the *ortho*-

lithiation of 1,4-dichlorobenzene **137** as the first reaction step [24]. Two lithium-mediated steps were required in this synthesis. The first lithium-mediated step was used to generate the triflouromethyl ketone derivative **142**. An optimum yield of 87% was obtained at a residence time of 4 minutes in Loop 1 and 13.3 minutes in Loop 2 (Fig. **9**). At 6 minutes' residence time in Loop 1 and 20 minutes in Loop 2, the yield decreased to 63%. The flow synthesis of **142** was therefore concluded to be time and temperature dependent.

The second lithium-mediated step was needed to effect alkynylation of **142** with cyclopropylacetylene **143** to yield propargylic alcohol **144**. In a very short reaction time of 3 minutes, (Loop 1; 60 s and Loop 2; 120 s), 93% conversion was achieved (Fig. **10**).

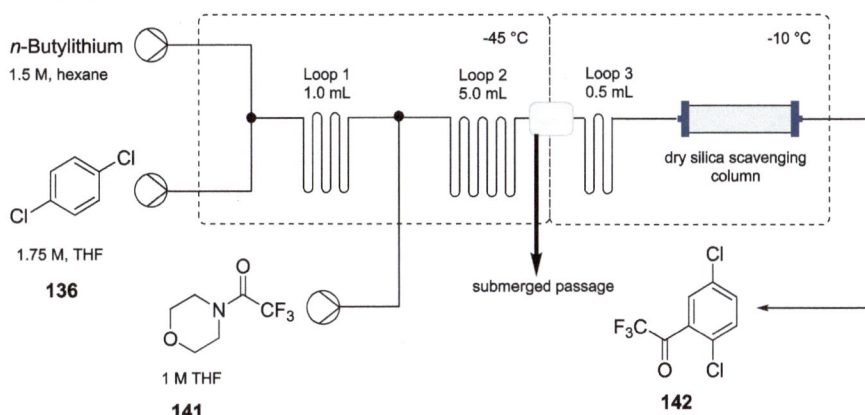

Fig. (9). Continuous flow synthesis of trifluoromethyl ketone derivative **142**.

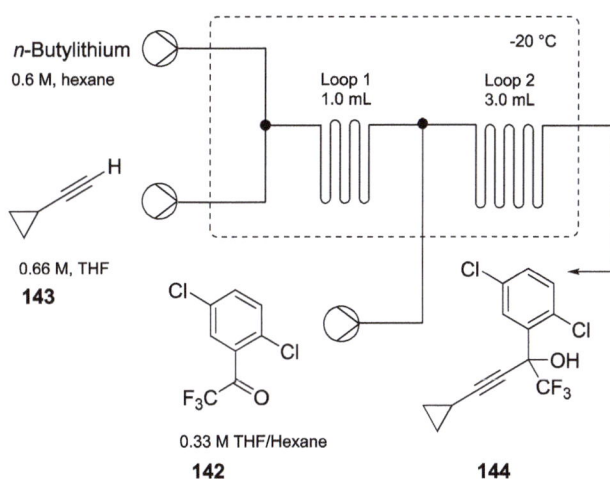

Fig. (10). Continuous flow alkynylation of 1-(2,5-dichlorophenyl)-2,2,2-trifluoroethan-1-one.

These two steps were successfully telescoped from which an isolated yield of 73% was obtained (0.5 mmol trifluoroacylating agent **141**, 0.5 M cyclopropylacetylene **143** and 0.43 M *n*-BuLi). After successfully synthesising intermediate **144**, the copper catalysed cyclization of an *in-situ* generated aryl isocyanate was investigated (Scheme **18**). A number of ligands and copper catalysts were meticulously investigated in the batch synthesis of Efavirenz **136** from propargylic alcohol **144**.

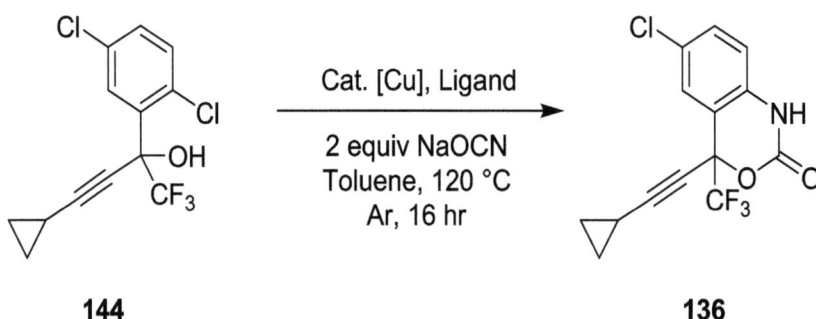

Scheme 18. Batch synthesis of Efavirenz from Propargylic alcohol **144**.

It was found that 20 mol % of CuSO$_4$ and Cu(NO$_3$)$_2$.3H$_2$O each used in combination with trans-*N,N*'-dimethyl-1,2-cyclohexanediamine (CyDMEDA), in a ratio of 1:4, gave satisfactory yields of **145**; 62% and 60% respectively. Additionally, the group were positive that in the flow synthesis, the formation of *ortho*-dechlorinated propargylic alcohol observed in the 16-hour batch synthesis would be curbed due to the assured accurate reaction parameter control in flow systems.

A preliminary flow experiment performed at 120 °C, (20:80 mol % of Cu(NO$_3$)$_2$.3H$_2$O and CyDMEDA respectively, 20 equiv NaOCN and 0.05 M alcohol **144**) in the above continuous flow reactor set up (Fig. **11**) at a flow rate of 33 µL/min, gave a 43% conversion and 19% yield of **136** at a residence time of 60 minutes. The low conversion was attributed to the slow reduction of Cu^{I} to Cu^{II}. On further investigation, with the aim of improving the product yield, it was found that the addition of Cu^0 powder accelerates both the reduction step and the oxidative addition of **144**. Unfortunately, this did not improve the yield of **136** since the transmetalation step is slow. It was also observed that a 1:2 catalyst to ligand ratio in addition to 1 equiv Cu^0, seemed to improve conversion of **144** to product **136** (32% yield) however, at such a low catalyst loading, there is a risk of the catalyst deactivating. This was circumvented by decreasing the NaOCN concentration and indeed at these conditions, 65% yield was attained (0.1 M alcohol, 1 equiv Cu^0, 5 mol % Cu(NO$_3$)$_2$.3H$_2$O and 10 mol % CyDMEDA).

$Cu(NO_3)_2.3H_2O$ was replaced with soluble $Cu(OTf)_2$ since at a 3:1 $PhCH_3$ to CH_3CN solvent system ratio, $Cu(NO_3)_2.3H_2O$ was insoluble at higher concentrations. From a 0.2 M concentration of alcohol **144**, 5 mol % $Cu(OTf)_2$, 10 mol % CyDMEDA, 0.5 equiv Cu^0 and 20 equiv NaOCN, 71% conversion of **144** and 61% isolated yield of Efavirenz **136** was obtained at 120 °C in only 60 minutes. It is of note that an overall yield of 45% was reported from the telescoped two-step synthesis of the propargyl alcohol **144** (Fig. **10**) and the one-step continuous flow synthesis of Efavirenz **136** from **144** (Fig. **11**). This was all achieved in less than 2 hours compared to the 16-hour batch synthesis.

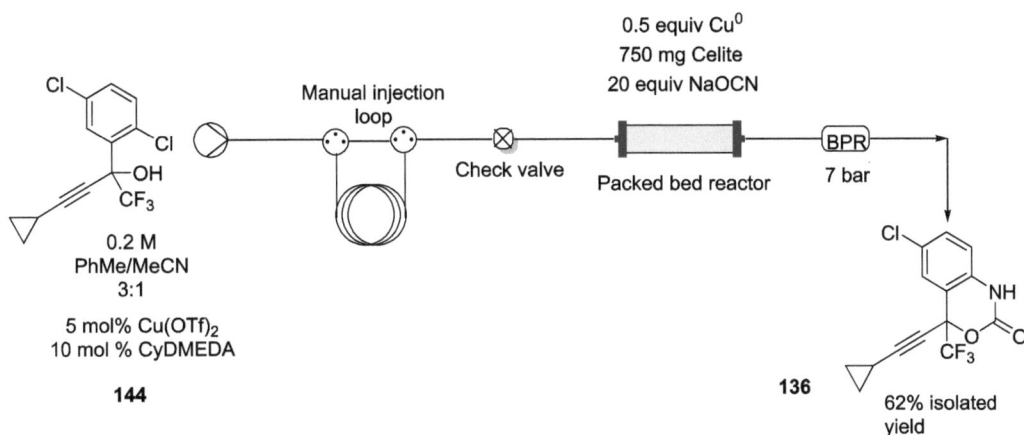

Fig. (11). Copper catalysed cyclization of an *in-situ* generated aryl isocyanate.

SEMI-CONTINUOUS FLOW SYNTHESIS OF LAMIVUDINE

Lamivudine **128** is a nucleoside reverse transcriptase inhibitor sold under trade names; Epivir and Epivir-HBV. It is reported to have high potency in the treatment of HIV-1 and Hepatisis B Virus as well as the Human T-Lymphotropic Virus (HTLV) [66, 67]. Mandala *et al.* report a semi-continuous flow synthesis of Lamivudine.(26) 5-acetoxy oxathiolane **149**, the first key intermediate, was synthesised in a two-step telescoped continuous flow synthesis beginning from menthyl glyoxalate **145** and 1,4-dithiane-2,5-diol **146** (Fig. **12**). The flow synthesis of intermediates **147** and **149** was first attempted individually in Little Things Factory microreactors prior to telescoping. 5-hydroxy oxathiolane **147** was obtained in 88% conversion in 20 minutes from **145** (0.43 M) and **146** (0.22 M) in acetonitrile that were pumped into a 2 mL reactor kept at 110 °C. To yield (2R,5R)-5-acetoxyoxathiolane **150**, 5-hydroxy oxathiolane **147** (0.34 M) was treated with acetic anhydride and pyridine (2.17 M) **148** in acetonitrile. The reaction step was carried out in a 1.9 mL reactor volume at ambient temperature to give a 95% conversion. A batch recrystallization of the crude at -20 °C gave isomer **150** in 48% yield. The authors achieved an optimum conversion of 95% in only 9.7 minutes from their telescoped two step synthesis.

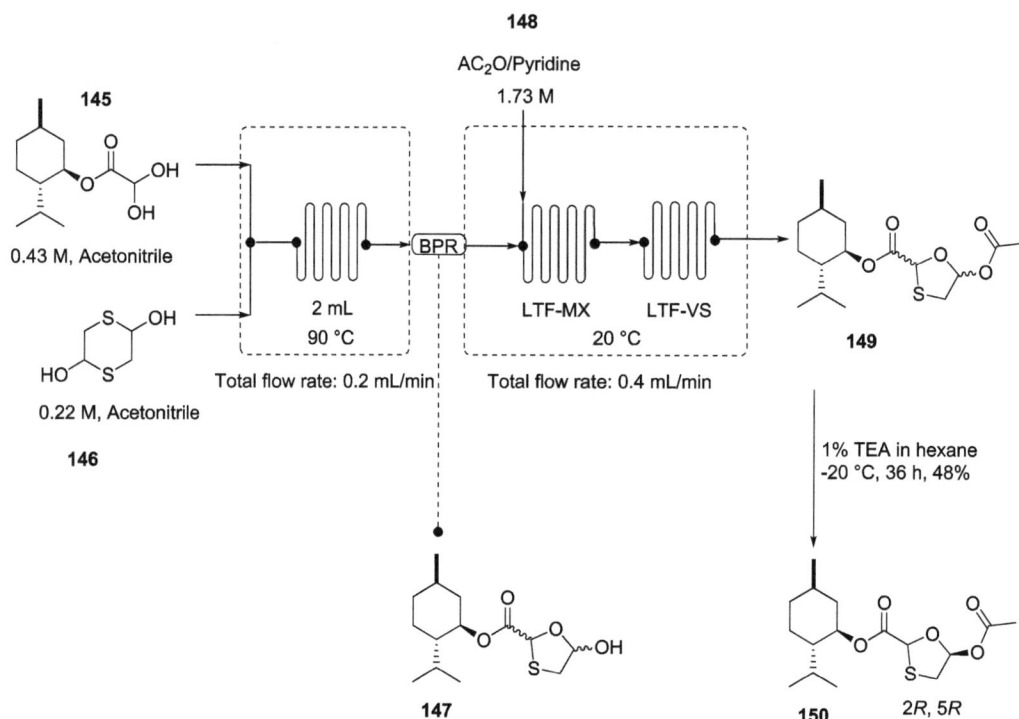

Fig. (12). Continuous flow synthesis of (2*R*,5*R*)-5-acetoxyoxathiolane.

The next step involved the *N*-glycosidation of isomer **150** with nucleobase **151** in the presence of pyridinium triflate. The poor solubility of the silylated nucleobase base however, which is not an issue in the batch *N*-glycosidation reaction, posed major challenges in flow. This was overcome with the use of thermal controlled syringe wrapping which maintained the nucleobase syringe solution at 55-60 °C throughout the experimentation (Fig. **13**). At 80 °C, the *N*-glycosidation product **152** was furnished in 95% yield in only 8.4 minutes. In such a short reaction time, a high yield was attained unlike in the batch synthesis. The flow synthesis also allowed for the use of a low catalyst concentration (0.2 M).

The reduction of nucleoside **152** to yield Lamuvidine **128** was carried out using NaBH$_4$ in the presence of K$_2$HPO$_4$ and was rapidly optimised in Little Things Factory microreactors (Fig. **14**). At a residence time of 3.3 minutes and reaction temperature of 20 °C, 100% conversion of **152** to **128** was achieved. The crude product was thereafter subjected to recrystallization from which 95% isolated yield with > 99% purity of **128** was obtained.

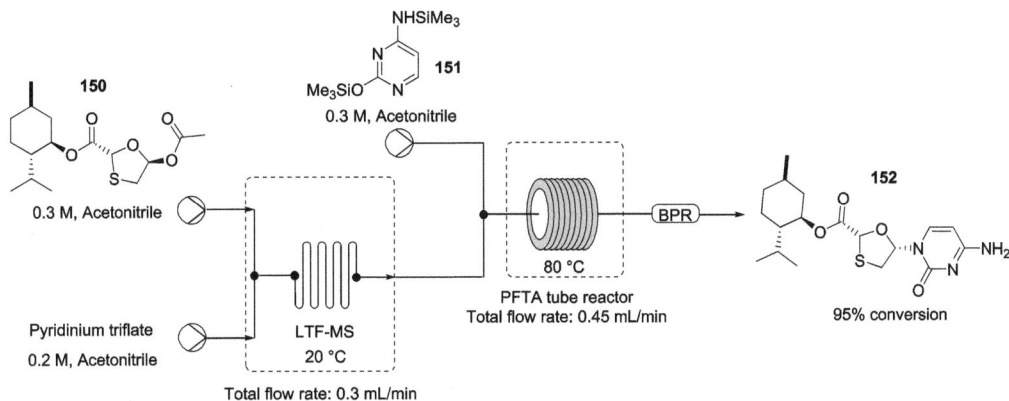

Fig. (13). Continuous flow *N*-glycosidation of (1*R*,2*S*,5*R*)-2-isopropyl-5-methylcyclohexyl (2*R*,5*R*)--acetoxy-1,3-oxathiolane-2-carboxylate **150**.

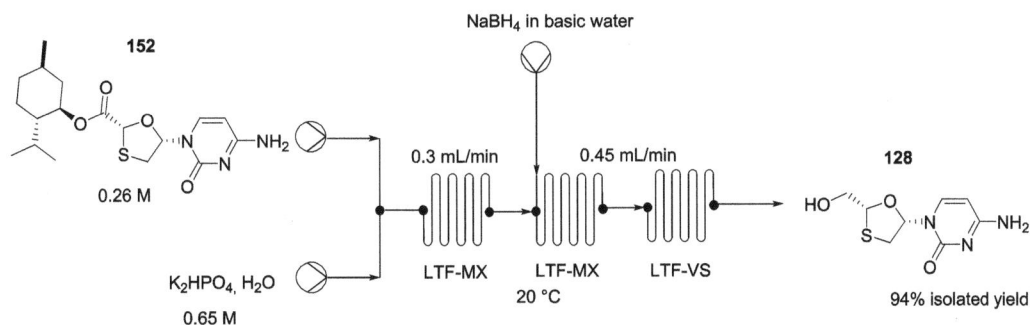

Fig. (14). Microreactor configuration for the reduction of nucleoside **152**.

CONTINUOUS FLOW SYNTHESIS OF INTERMEDIATES TOWARDS DARUNAVIR AND ATAZANIVIR

A three-step continuous flow synthesis of a non-peptidal bis-tetrahydrofuran moiety of Darunavir **153**, another important compound for HIV treatment, has recently been reported [28]. As is common with most reports demonstrating the advantages of continuous flow processing for API synthesis, preliminary studies were carried out in batch to better understand the reaction (Scheme **19**).

The synthesis of (3*R*,3*aS*,6*aR*)-hexahydrofuro[2,3-b]furan-3-ol (-)-**158**, was started from the ozonolysis of (3*aS*,6*aR*)-3-methylenehexahydrofuro[2,3-b]furan (+/-)-**154**. Using an IceCube™ flow reactor with an ozone module at -30 °C, 99% yield (3*aR*,6*aR*)-tetrahydrofuro[2,3-b]furan-3(2*H*)-one (+/-)-**155** was recorded in only 4 minutes. This is a much shorter reaction time compared to the 3 hours required to achieve comparable yield in the batch synthesis. The first attempt towards a continuous flow reduction of (+/-)-**155** was effected with BH$_4$

immobilised on Amberlyst at room temperature. This provided racemic alcohol (+/-)-**156** in 91% isolated yield in 30 minutes. The continuous flow process gave a space-time yield of 1239 g/L/day (Fig. **15**). This was further improved by employing 5% Ru/C catalysed hydrogenation using an H-Cube Pro™ system. In a residence time of 1.39 minutes at 75 °C, a space-time yield of 6.7 g/L/day was obtained. The batch kinetic resolution of (+/-)-**156** was similarly translated into a continuous flow process which provided better conversion in a short amount of time. In a nutshell, the flow synthesis of (-)-**156**, provided better space-time yield. 1.2 kg of alcohol per litre per day compared to 0.69 kg obtained from the batch synthesis (Fig. **15**). The advantages of translating the three step batch synthesis of intermediate (-)-**158** towards Darunavir, into continuous flow syntheses, were unequivocally demonstrated.

de Souza *et al.* recently reported a three step continuous flow synthesis of a biaryl unit of an HIV protease inhibitor, Atazanavir **160** [27]. The flow synthesis consisted of a Suzuki Mayaura coupling of 4-formyl-phenylboronic acid **161** and

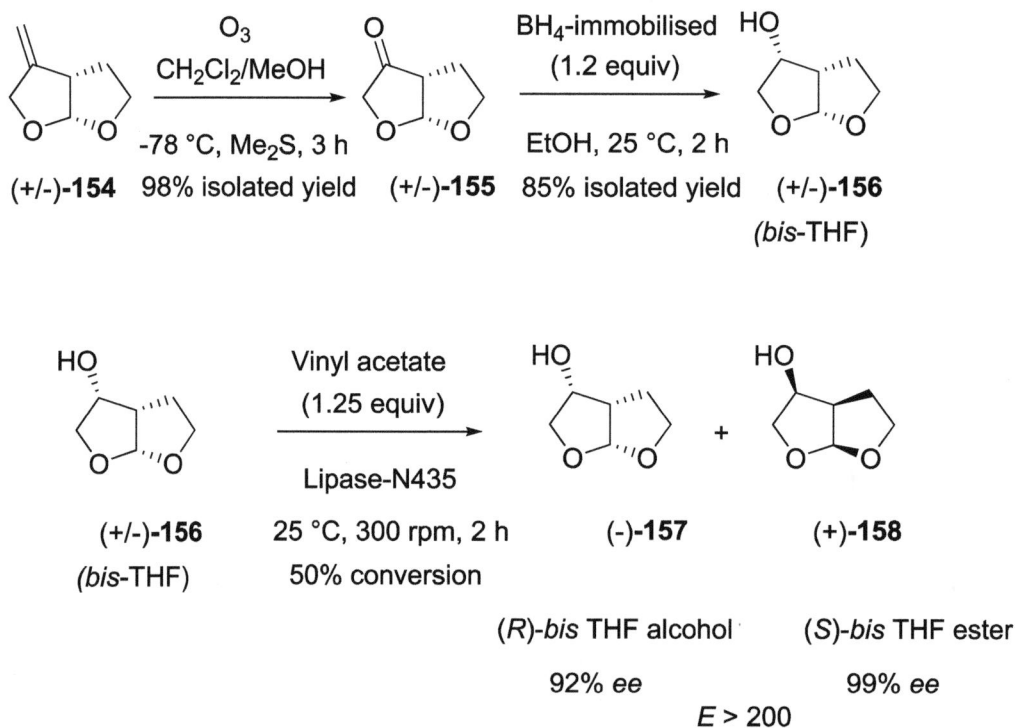

Scheme 19. Batch synthesis of (3*R*,3a*S*,6a*R*)-hexahydrofuro[2,3-b]furan-3-ol.

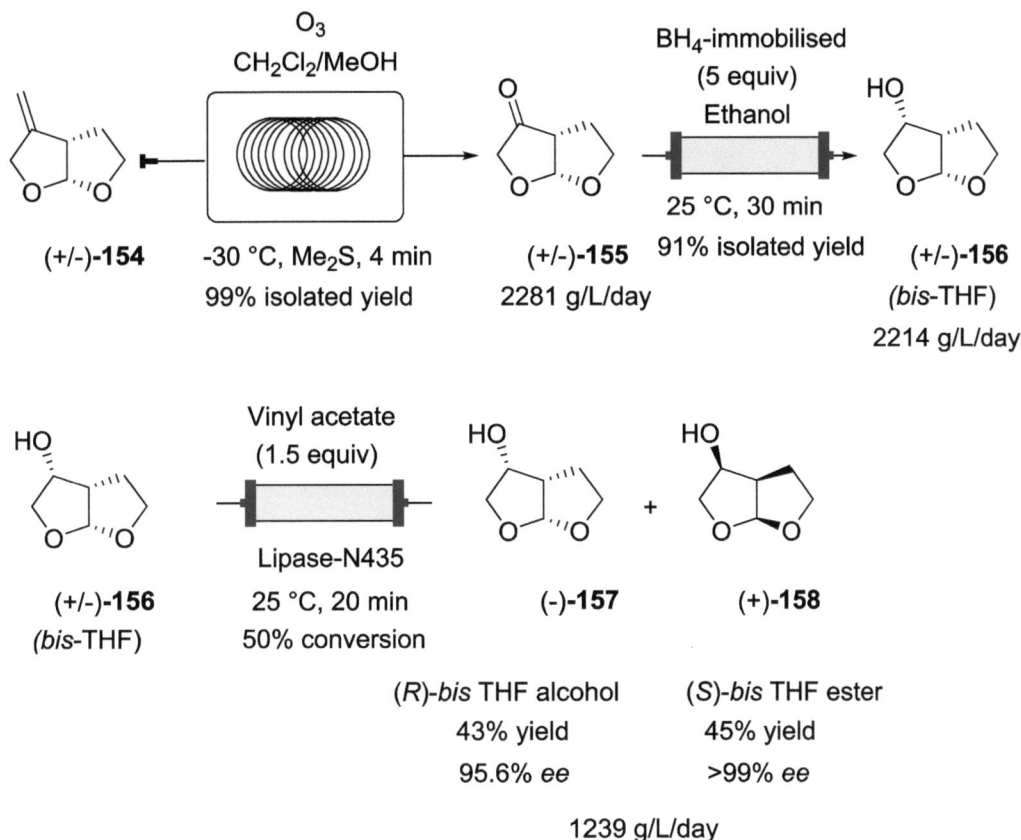

Fig. (15). Continuous flow synthesis of (3*R*,3*aS*,6*aR*)-hexahydrofuro[2,3-*b*]furan-3-ol.

2-bromo pyridine **162** under phase transfer conditions in a 4 mL stainless steel reactor (0.02 inch i.d.) (Fig. **16**). At 150 °C, 95% conversion to biaryl compound **163** was achieved in 20 minutes. From prior batch microwave synthesis of hydrazone **165**, it was found that crude biaryl compound **163** could be used. The two reaction steps; Suzuki Mayaura and hydrazone formation were thus optimised and telescoped in a Syrris Asia flow system. A 99% conversion was achieved in 8 minutes at 50 °C from crude **163** (0.1 M) and tert-butyl carbazate **164** (1.2 equiv) in the presence of trimethylsilytriflate (0.75 equiv). A liquid-liquid extractor was employed to eliminate the acid from the hydrazone formation and in so doing, the crude hydrazone effluent was made suitable for the next reaction step *i.e.* hydrogenation. As a result, the three reaction steps were telescoped in a continuous flow process to give compound **166** in an overall yield of 74% after chromatography purification.

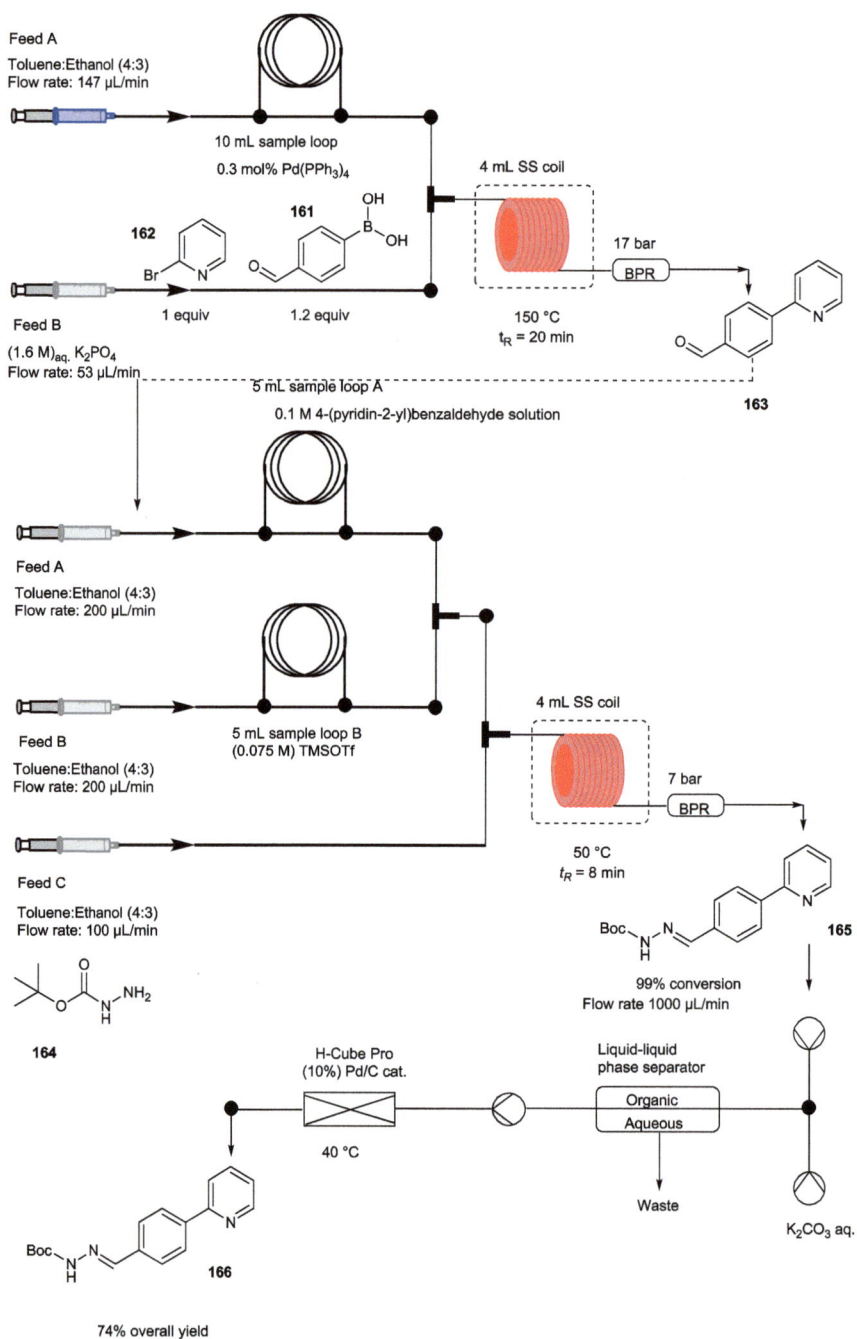

Fig. (16). Continuous flow synthesis of a biaryl unit of Atazanavir.

Kappe *et al.* developed a multi-step continuous flow process for the synthesis of α-chloro ketone **170**, an important building block towards the synthesis of Darunavir **153** and Atazanavir **160** [68]. The intermediate was obtained from diazomethane, which was generated *in-situ*. The continuous flow system enabled the safe *in-situ* generation and use of diazomethane to afford batch chemistries involving its use. The use of diazomethane is rarely explored due to the safety risks involved. It is very volatile and delicate in nature (boiling point -23 °C). It is also toxic yet odourless moreover, if subjected to abrupt change in temperature, is explosive. Cbz protected *L*-phenylalanine **167** was activated with ethyl chloroformate **168** in the presence of tributylamine at room temperature to form an anhydride in 6.7 minutes. The diazomethane formed from Diazald **169** in the tube in tube reactor, was thereafter immediately reacted with the anhydride for 31.7 minutes at room temperature to form the corresponding α-diazo ketone. This was subjected to an ethereal solution of HCl in diethyl ether at 0 °C in turn affording 87% of desired α-chloro ketone **170**, a key intermediate for the synthesis of protease inhibitors, Darunavir and Atazanavir (Fig. **17**).

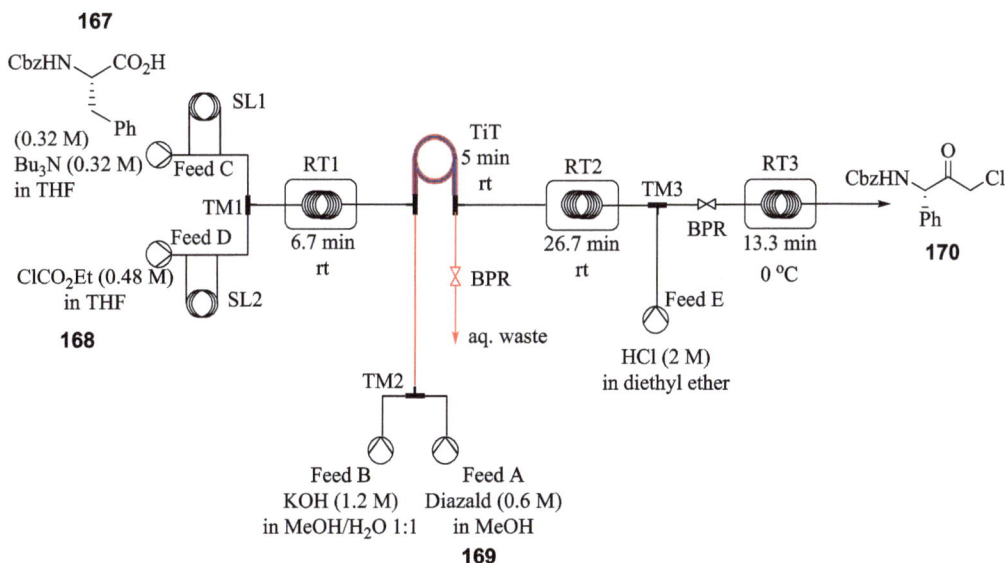

Fig. (17). Continuous flow synthesis of α-chloro ketone, a Darunavir and Atazanavir key intermediate.

The continuous flow syntheses of the above discussed HIV drugs and APIs clearly demonstrate the numerous benefits of translating batch syntheses into continuous flow processes. As such, this should be a motivating factor for further investigative research at laboratory level as well as garnering possible collaborations with the industrial players.

CONCLUSION

HIV/AIDS is evidently a global health burden however; credit should be given to the tremendous efforts put in to combat the disease. Since the discovery of the virus, the emergence of INSTIs *i.e.* first and second generation anti HIV drugs has been witnessed. The synthesis and development of these drug APIs can also be said to have evolved. Their synthesis, although is still predominantly based on traditional batch methods, is steadily moving towards the more cost effective, high yielding continuous flow synthesis approach. Notably, the support from the FDA is the driving factor for the advancement in the application of different synthetic protocols used in the development of INSTIs. This represents a major breakthrough in the history of HIV Drug research. The safe, efficacious and well tolerated; Dolutegravir and Bictegravir with high resistance profile, present a unique characteristic in the history of ART. Moreover, with the introduction of continuous flow processing to HIV drug and API manufacture, we foresee a shorter time to market and a boost in affordability as well as accessibility of these important compounds to regions and persons in need.

CONSENT FOR PUBLICATION

Not applicable.

CONFLICT OF INTEREST

The author (editor) declares no conflict of interest, financial or otherwise.

ACKNOWLEDGEMENTS

We would like to thank the Nelson Mandela University and the National Research Foundation South Africa for their financial support.

REFERENCES

[1]   Silverman RB. The Organic Chemistry of Drug Design and Drug Action. 2nd ed., San Diego: Elsevier Academic Press 2004.

[2]   Li JJ, Johnson DS, Sliskovic DR, Roth BD. Contemporary Drug Synthesis. John Wiley and Sons 2004.
        [http://dx.doi.org/10.1002/0471686743]

[3]   Nicolaou KC. Organic synthesis: The art and science of replicating the molecules of living nature and creating others like them in the laboratory. Proc R Soc A Math Phys Eng Sci 2014; 470(2163): 1-171.

[4]   Nicolaou KC, Montagnon T. Molecules that Changed the World. Wiley-VCH 2008.

[5]   Walensky RP, Paltiel AD, Losina E, *et al.* The survival benefits of AIDS treatment in the United States. J Infect Dis 2006; 194(1): 11-9.
        [http://dx.doi.org/10.1086/505147] [PMID: 16741877]

[6]   Trezza C, Ford SL, Spreen W, Pan R, Piscitelli S. Formulation and pharmacology of long-acting

cabotegravir. Curr Opin HIV AIDS 2015; 10(4): 239-45.
[http://dx.doi.org/10.1097/COH.0000000000000168]

[7]   UNAIDS. UNAIDS Global statistics 2018 [Internet] 2018 Available from: http://wwwunaidsorg /sites /default /files /media_asset/UNAIDS_FactSheet_enpdf

[8]   Arts EJ, Hazuda DJ, Bushman EFD, Nabel GJ, Swanstrom R. HIV-1 antiretroviral drug therapy. Cold Spring Harb Perspect Med 2012; 2(4): a007161.
[http://dx.doi.org/10.1101/cshperspect.a007161] [PMID: 22474613]

[9]   Maurin C, Bailly F, Cotelle P. Structure-activity relationships of HIV-1 integrase inhibitors--enzye-ligand interactions. Curr Med Chem 2003; 10(18): 1795-810.
[http://dx.doi.org/10.2174/0929867033456981] [PMID: 12871105]

[10]   Lesbats P, Engelman AN, Cherepanov P. Retroviral DNA Integration. Chem Rev 2016; 116(20): 12730-57.
[http://dx.doi.org/10.1021/acs.chemrev.6b00125] [PMID: 27198982]

[11]   Hazuda DJ, Felock P, Witmer M, *et al.* Inhibitors of strand transfer that prevent integration and inhibit HIV-1 replication in cells. Science 2000; 287(5453): 646-50.
[http://dx.doi.org/10.1126/science.287.5453.646] [PMID: 10649997]

[12]   Guidelines for the Use of Antiretroviral Agents in Pediatric HIV Infection [Internet] Panel on Antiretroviral Therapy and Medical Managemaent of Children Living with HIV 2018 [cited 2018 Jun 19] p M136–60 Available from: http://aidsinfonihgov/con-tentfiles/Ivguidelines/pediatric guidelinespdf

[13]   Dow DE, Bartlett JA. Dolutegravir, the Second-Generation of Integrase Strand Transfer Inhibitors (INSTIs) for the Treatment of HIV. Infect Dis Ther 2014; 3(2): 83-102.
[http://dx.doi.org/10.1007/s40121-014-0029-7] [PMID: 25134686]

[14]   Blanco JL, Whitlock G, Milinkovic A, Moyle G. HIV integrase inhibitors: a new era in the treatment of HIV. Expert Opin Pharmacother 2015; 16(9): 1313-24.
[http://dx.doi.org/10.1517/14656566.2015.1044436] [PMID: 26001181]

[15]   Summa V, Petrocchi A, Bonelli F, *et al.* Discovery of raltegravir, a potent, selective orally bioavailable HIV-integrase inhibitor for the treatment of HIV-AIDS infection. J Med Chem 2008; 51(18): 5843-55.
[http://dx.doi.org/10.1021/jm800245z] [PMID: 18763751]

[16]   Gupta A, Juneja S, Vitoria M, *et al.* Projected uptake of new antiretroviral (ARV) medicines in adults in low- and middle-income countries: A forecast analysis 2015-2025. PLoS One 2016; 11(10): e0164619.
[http://dx.doi.org/10.1371/journal.pone.0164619] [PMID: 27736953]

[17]   Baxendale IR, Hayward JJ, Ley SV, Tranmer GK. Pharmaceutical strategy and innovation: an academics perspective. ChemMedChem 2007; 2(6): 768-88.
[http://dx.doi.org/10.1002/cmdc.200700008] [PMID: 17458911]

[18]   https://medicines4all.vcu.edu./

[19]   Longstreet AR, Opalka SM, Campbell BS, Gupton BF, McQuade DT. Investigating the continuous synthesis of a nicotinonitrile precursor to nevirapine. Beilstein J Org Chem 2013; 9: 2570-8.
[http://dx.doi.org/10.3762/bjoc.9.292] [PMID: 24367421]

[20]   De Souza ROMA, Watts P. Flow Processing as a Tool for API Production in Developing Economies. J Flow Chem 2017; 7(October): 146-50.
[http://dx.doi.org/10.1556/1846.2017.00019]

[21]   Movsisyan M, Delbeke EIP, Berton JKET, Battilocchio C, Ley SV, Stevens CV. Taming hazardous chemistry by continuous flow technology. Chem Soc Rev 2016; 45(18): 4892-928.
[http://dx.doi.org/10.1039/C5CS00902B] [PMID: 27453961]

[22] Mcwilliams JC, Allian AD, Opalka SM, May SA, Journet M, Braden TM. The Evolving State of Continuous Processing in Pharmaceutical API Manufacturing: A Survey of Pharmaceutical Companies and Contract Manufacturing Organizations. Org Process Res Dev 2018; 22: 1143-66.
[http://dx.doi.org/10.1021/acs.oprd.8b00160]

[23] Ziegler RE, Bimbisar K, Desai JJ, Gupton BF, Roper TD, Jamison TF. 7-Step Flow Synthesis of the HIV Integrase Inhibitor Dolutegravir Zuschriften Angewandte. Angew Chem Int Ed 2018; 130: 7299-303.
[http://dx.doi.org/10.1002/ange.201802256]

[24] Correia CA, Gilmore K, McQuade DT, Seeberger PH. A concise flow synthesis of efavirenz. Angew Chem Int Ed Engl 2015; 54(16): 4945-8.
[http://dx.doi.org/10.1002/anie.201411728] [PMID: 25727078]

[25] Chada S, Mandala D, Watts P. Synthesis of a Key Intermediate towards the Preparation of Efavirenz Using n -Butyllithium. J Flow Chem 2017; 7: 37-40.
[http://dx.doi.org/10.1556/1846.2017.00008]

[26] Mandala D, Chada S, Watts P. Semi-continuous multi-step synthesis of lamivudine. Org Biomol Chem 2017; 15(16): 3444-54.
[http://dx.doi.org/10.1039/C7OB00480J] [PMID: 28362445]

[27] Dalla-Vechia L, Reichart B, Glasnov T, Miranda LSM, Kappe CO, de Souza RO. A three step continuous flow synthesis of the biaryl unit of the HIV protease inhibitor Atazanavir. Org Biomol Chem 2013; 11(39): 6806-13.
[http://dx.doi.org/10.1039/C3OB41464G] [PMID: 24175328]

[28] Leão RAC, Lopes R de O, Bezerra MA de M, Muniz MN, Casanova BB, SCB Gnoatto. Studies on the continuous-flow synthesis of nonpeptidal bis-tetrahydrofuran moiety of Darunavir. J Flow Chem 2015; 5(4): 216-9.

[29] Pharmaceutical Technology Editors. FDA Approves Tablet Production on Janssen Continuous Manufacturing Line [Internet] 2016 [cited 2018 Sep 10] Available from: http://wwwpharmtechcom /fda- approves- tablet- production- janssen- continuous-manufacturing-line

[30] Marriott N. EMA approves Janssen's Prezista continuous manufacturing line [Internet] European Pharmaceutical Review 2017 [cited 2018 Sep 12] Available from: http://wwwpharmtechcom /ema-approves- janssen- drug- made- continuous-manufacturing

[31] Grobler JA, Stillmock K, Hu B, *et al.* Diketo acid inhibitor mechanism and HIV-1 integrase: implications for metal binding in the active site of phosphotransferase enzymes. Proc Natl Acad Sci USA 2002; 99(10): 6661-6.
[http://dx.doi.org/10.1073/pnas.092056199] [PMID: 11997448]

[32] Croxtall JD, Scott LJ. Raltegravir: in treatment-naive patients with HIV-1 infection. Drugs 2010; 70(5): 631-42.
[http://dx.doi.org/10.2165/11204590-000000000-00000] [PMID: 20329808]

[33] Nguyen BYT, Isaacs RD, Teppler H, *et al.* Raltegravir: the first HIV-1 integrase strand transfer inhibitor in the HIV armamentarium. Ann N Y Acad Sci 2011; 1222(1): 83-9.
[http://dx.doi.org/10.1111/j.1749-6632.2011.05972.x] [PMID: 21434946]

[34] Teppler H. Long-Term Safety from the Raltegravir Clinical Development Program Curr HIV Res [Internet] 2011;9(1):40–53 Available from: http://wwweurekaselectcom /openurl /content php? genre= article&issn=1570-162X&volume=9&issue=1&spage=40

[35] Deeks ED. Raltegravir Once-Daily Tablet: A Review in HIV-1 Infection. Drugs 2017; 77(16): 1789-95.
[http://dx.doi.org/10.1007/s40265-017-0827-9] [PMID: 29071467]

[36] Humphrey GR, Pye PJ, Zhong YL, Angelaud R, Askin D, Belyk KM, *et al.* Development of a second-generation, highly efficient manufacturing route for the HIV integrase inhibitor raltegravir potassium.

Org Process Res Dev 2011; 15(1): 73-83.
[http://dx.doi.org/10.1021/op100257r]

[37]   Mukund K G, Swapnil P S, Golakchandra S M, *et al.* Samit SM. Synthesis of raltegravir WO 2013098854 A2 2013.

[38]   Clavel F. HIV resistance to raltegravir. Eur J Med Res 2009; 14 (Suppl. 3): 47-54.
[http://dx.doi.org/10.1186/2047-783X-14-S3-47] [PMID: 19959417]

[39]   Satoh M, Kawakami H, Itoh Y, *et al.* Al E 4-Oxoquinoline Compounds and Utilization thereof as HIV Integrase Inhibitors 2004 p 1–166.

[40]   Sato M, Motomura T, Aramaki H, *et al.* Novel HIV-1 integrase inhibitors derived from quinolone antibiotics. J Med Chem 2006; 49(5): 1506-8.
[http://dx.doi.org/10.1021/jm0600139] [PMID: 16509568]

[41]   Wainberg MA, Mesplède T, Quashie PK. The development of novel HIV integrase inhibitors and the problem of drug resistance. Curr Opin Virol 2012; 2(5): 656-62.
[http://dx.doi.org/10.1016/j.coviro.2012.08.007] [PMID: 22989757]

[42]   Matsuda K, Ando K, Ohki SH. Compound US 8,383,819 B2 2013

[43]   Dowdy E, Chen X, Pfeiffer S. Process and Intermediates for Preparing Integrase Inhibitors US 8324244B2 2012

[44]   Radi S. An Improved Production Method and New Intermediates of Synthesis of Elvitegravir WO 2014; 2014/056465: A1.

[45]   Anstett K, Brenner B, Mesplede T, Wainberg MA. HIV drug resistance against strand transfer integrase inhibitors. Retrovirology 2017; 14(1): 36.
[http://dx.doi.org/10.1186/s12977-017-0360-7] [PMID: 28583191]

[46]   Reddy Shankar B. An I mproved Process for the Preparation of Dolutegravir W014/1284545A2 2014

[47]   Johns BA. The Polycyclic CarbamoylPyridone Derivative Having Hiv Integrase Inhibitory Activity WO 2006/116764A1

[48]   Sumino Y, Masui M, Yamada D, Ikarashi F, Okamoto K. Method of Producing Pyrone and Pyridone derivatives US 2014/0011995 A1 2014

[49]   Yukihito S, Kazuya O, Moriyasu M, Daisuke Y, Fumiya I. Process for preparing compound having hiv integrase inhibitory activity EP 2602260 A1 2013

[50]   Wang H, Goodman SV, Mann D KM. The Process for Preparing Carbamoylpyridone Derivatives and Intermediates WO 2011/119566 2014

[51]   Sankareswaran S, Mannam M, Chakka V, Mandapati SR, Kumar P. Identi fi cation and Control of Critical Process Impurities: An Improved Process for the Preparation of Dolutegravir Sodium. Org Process Res Dev 2016; 20: 1461-8.
[http://dx.doi.org/10.1021/acs.oprd.6b00156]

[52]   Gilead Sciences I. (NASDAQ:GILD US Food and Drug Administration Approves Gilead's Biktarvy® (Bictegravir, Emtricitabine, Tenofovir Alafenamide) for Treatment of HIV-1 Infection FOSTER CITY, Calif--(BUSINESS WIRE) 2018

[53]   Jin H, Lazerwith SE, Trejo Martin T. Polycyclic Carbamoylpyridone Compounds and their Pharmaceutical Use US 2006 / 0222585 A1 2006

[54]   Lancster M. Green Chemistry; An Introductory Text.Designing Greener Processes. 3rd ed. Cambridge: The Royal Society of Chemistry, Thomas Graham House, Science Park, Milton Road 2002; pp. 235-40.

[55]   Lee SL, O'Connor TF, Yang X, Cruz CN, Chatterjee S, Yu LX, *et al.* Modernizing Pharmaceutical Manufacturing : from Batch to Continuous Production. J Pharm Innov 2015; 10: 191-9.
[http://dx.doi.org/10.1007/s12247-015-9215-8]

[56]   Plumb K. Continuous processing in the pharmaceutical industry Changing the Mind Set. Chem Eng Res Des 2005; 83(A6): 730-8.
[http://dx.doi.org/10.1205/cherd.04359]

[57]   Kaeding P. Pharmaceutical cGMPS for the 21st Century-A Risk Based Approach Philadelphia; 2005.

[58]   Hughes DL. Applications of Flow Chemistry in Drug Development: Highlights of Recent Patent Literature. Org Process Res Dev 2018; 22: 13-20.
[http://dx.doi.org/10.1021/acs.oprd.7b00363]

[59]   Gérardy R, Emmanuel N, Toupy T, *et al.* Continuous Flow Organic Chemistry : Successes and Pitfalls at the Interface with Current Societal Challenges 2018; 2301–51

[60]   Wiles C, Watts P. Green Chemistry Continuous flow reactors : a perspective 2012;38–54

[61]   Zhang P, Russell MG, Jamison TF. Continuous flow total synthesis of rufinamide. Org Process Res Dev 2014; 18(11): 1567-70.
[http://dx.doi.org/10.1021/op500166n]

[62]   Snead DR, Jamison TF. A Three-Minute Synthesis and Purification of Ibuprofen : Pushing the Limits of Continuous-Flow Processing ** Angewandte 2015; 983–7

[63]   Gilmore K, Kopetzki D, Lee JW, *et al.* Continuous synthesis of artemisinin-derived medicines. Chem Commun (Camb) 2014; 50(84): 12652-5.
[http://dx.doi.org/10.1039/C4CC05098C] [PMID: 25204815]

[64]   FDA-Approved HIV Medicines p https://wwwhhsgov/

[65]   De Clercq E. The role of non-nucleoside reverse transcriptase inhibitors (NNRTIs) in the therapy of HIV-1 infection. Antiviral Res 1998; 38(3): 153-79.
[http://dx.doi.org/10.1016/S0166-3542(98)00025-4] [PMID: 9754886]

[66]   Cihlar T, Ray AS. Nucleoside and nucleotide HIV reverse transcriptase inhibitors: 25 years after zidovudine. Antiviral Res 2010; 85(1): 39-58.
[http://dx.doi.org/10.1016/j.antiviral.2009.09.014] [PMID: 19887088]

[67]   Férir G, Kaptein S, Neyts J, De Clercq E. Antiviral treatment of chronic hepatitis B virus infections: the past, the present and the future. Rev Med Virol 2008; 18(1): 19-34.
[http://dx.doi.org/10.1002/rmv.554] [PMID: 17966115]

[68]   Pinho VD, Gutmann B, Miranda LSM, de Souza ROMA, Kappe CO. Continuous flow synthesis of α-halo ketones: essential building blocks of antiretroviral agents. J Org Chem 2014; 79(4): 1555-62.
[http://dx.doi.org/10.1021/jo402849z] [PMID: 24471789]

The Development and Clinical Progress on Chemokine Receptor-Based HIV Entry Inhibitors

Yi-Qun Kuang[*]

Center for Translational Medicine, Huaihe Clinical College, Huaihe Hospital of Henan University, Kaifeng, Henan, China

Abstract: Entry of HIV-1 into targeted host cells is a highly ordered multistage process involving first-receptor attachment, co-receptor binding, and membrane fusion. In this chapter, I will present an overview of progress on HIV-1 entry inhibitors with a focus on chemokine receptor-based antagonists. This chapter, at first, will describe the working mechanisms of chemokine receptors, HIV-1 co-receptors CCR5 and CXCR4, during the replication procedure. Then, the antagonists-based on different mechanisms will be presented in detail. At last, it will summarize and explain the distinct promising entry inhibitors based on co-receptors-interacting proteins, which is inspired by our current work.

Keywords: AIDS, CCR5, Chemokine receptor, Co-receptor, CXCR4, Entry inhibitor, HIV.

INTRODUCTION

The application of potent combination antiretroviral therapy (cART), also called highly active antiretroviral therapy (HAART), has considerably reduced the morbidity and mortality from Human immunodeficiency virus type 1 (HIV-1) infection over the world. To date, there are 28 FDA-approved drugs targeting the HIV-1 lifecycle, including one Entry Inhibitor (EI), one Fusion Inhibitor (FI), three Integrase Inhibitors (INI), four Non-nucleoside Reverse Transcriptase Inhibitors (NNRTI), 10 Nucleoside Reverse Transcriptase Inhibitors (NRTI), and 9 Protease Inhibitors (PI). In addition, there are 14 Combination Drugs, 50 drugs for Opportunistic Infections and Coinfections, and one Pharmacokinetic Enhancers (CYP3A Inhibitors) approved for treatment of HIV/AIDS infection and complications. Among them, the three major classes (NRTI, NNRTI, and PI) target two HIV-1-replication-dependent enzymes, reverse transcriptase and

[*] **Corresponding author Yi-Qun Kuang:** Center for Translational Medicine, Huaihe Clinical College, Huaihe Hospital of Henan University, Kaifeng, Henan, China; Tel: (86-371) 23906991; Fax: (86-371) 23906888; E-mail: yqkuang@henu.edu.cn

Atta-ur-Rahman (Ed.)

protease. Although potent viral inhibition in HIV-infected patients can be achieved by treating with cART regimens, the occurrence or acquisition of drug-resistant HIV-1 strains results in treatment failure, and this can significantly limit the therapeutic options in the future [1]. Besides, use of HAART drugs results in a variety of adverse effects, which may significantly affect the continuation of medication in patients [1, 2]. In efforts to provide more therapeutic options to patients with drug-resistant strains or to support treatment with lower toxicities than existing therapies, a new class of drugs targeting HIV-1 entry into cells and possessing potent antiretroviral activity is being developed.

HIV-1 infects a cell through ways that fuse membrane and release its nucleocapsid (NC) core into the host cell [3]. The viral envelop glycoprotein (Env), a viral surface protein, consists of gp120 which offers the binding sites for the first receptor CD4, and gp41 that facilitates the fusion between Env and the host membrane, implying the significance of Env in receptor attachment and membrane fusion [4, 5]. In 1997, scientists found that the C-C chemokine receptor type 5 (CCR5) was the predominant co-receptor for HIV in early infection of R5-tropic cells, while the C-X-C chemokine receptor type 4 (CXCR4) was used later when the X4-tropic (HIV-1 strains that bind to CXCR4) emerged with disease progression [6, 7]. The entry process relies on the gp120 binding to CD4 receptor and subsequent binding to one of the co-receptors, either CCR5 or CXCR4. The CD4 binding results in conformational changes in gp120 and the sequential rapid exposure of the co-receptor binding site, and then triggers membrane fusion [8, 9]. The HIV-1 co-receptors CCR5 and CXCR4 belong to the G protein-coupled receptors (GPCRs) family. The global epidemic HIV-1 strains are CCR5 co-receptor tropic.

Although HAART is an effective measure for HIV-1 treatment, it is not capable of eradicating the virus from the human body [10]. The chemokine receptor antagonists, a new drug class, target cellular membrane proteins that serve as co-receptors for HIV-1 infection on the surface of $CD4^+$ T cells or macrophages, thereby blocking the interaction between the co-receptor and the viral envelope glycoprotein (gp120). Chemokine receptor antagonists are able to block the interaction between the HIV-1 envelope and CCR5 or CXCR4, thus potently inhibit HIV-1 replication *in vitro*. Pilot studies on orally bioavailable small-molecule CCR5 inhibitors in HIV-1-infected subjects have provided proof of concept for this novel drug class, and contributed to the first CCR5-based entry inhibitor in market. Now, a couple of new generation CCR5 antagonists at phase I-III safety and efficacy clinical trials are under way. Taking into account the co-receptors' critical role in HIV-1 infection, many HIV researchers hope to control HIV-1 infection through inhibiting the co-receptors binding to gp120 to prevent the virus from entering target cells. In recent years, scientists have made some progress in studying chemokine receptor antagonists, especially for CCR5. Maraviroc is the first FDA-approved CCR5 antagonist drug [11, 12]. PRO140, a humanized monoclonal antibody, binds to CCR5 and has potent antiviral activity in patients infected with R5-tropic viruses (HIV-1 strains that bind to CCR5) [13, 14]. Last year, Giroud *et al.* presented that NF279 can block the interaction between virus with both CCR5 and CXCR4, which therefore, was regarded as a dual HIV-1 co-receptor inhibitor [15]. All of these examples have demonstrated that the co-receptors-based inhibitors are a promising direction for anti-HIV-1 drug development. In this chapter, we will present the advances in CCR5-based HIV entry inhibitors and the mechanisms involved in detail.

In this chapter, I review the structure and biological function of CCR5 and CXCR4 in HIV-1 infection, and clarify the signal cascades activated by the co-receptors and their roles during viral entry and intracellular replication. I summarize the updating clinical data on the administration of chemokine co-receptor-based antagonists in treatment-naive and -experienced AIDS patients, and discuss the challenges posed during the clinical development of these novel inhibitors. I also present the emerging concerns and future perspectives on the chemokine receptor blockades, which derived from the molecules involved in the signaling assembly and signal transduction that elicited by HIV-1 glycoprotein *via* co-receptor. With this body of evidence in mind, I assess the potential role the chemokine receptor antagonists may play in cART against HIV-1 in the future.

I. THE ROLE OF HIV-1 CO-RECEPTORS IN VIRAL REPLICATION

The chemokine receptors CCR5 and CXCR4 are indispensable entry cofactors in HIV-1 infection. They are essential for membrane fusion. Both of them are G-protein coupled receptors with a hydrophobic pocket consisting of seven transmembrane helices [4, 16, 17]. HIV strains named R5-tropic interact with CD4 and CCR5, infect $CCR5^+$ $CD4^+$ T cell. The other viral strains which interact with CD4 and CXCR4, infect $CXCR4^+$ $CD4^+$ T cells and are called X4-tropic. R5-tropic preponderate in the early infection stages, while X4-tropic emerge in later stages and are considered as one reason accelerating AIDS progression, so CCR5 and CXCR4 clearly play different roles in the infection of HIV [18]. Some dual tropism viral strains are able to use both CCR5 and CXCR4 (termed R5/X4 viruses). Mixtures of R5-tropic and X4-tropic viruses are also found in patients. The commonly used tropism assays cannot distinguish dual-tropic virus from a mixture of R5-tropic and X4-tropic viruses, thus such samples are referred to as dual-mixed (D/M)-tropic viruses. CXCR4 may interact with Env directly or involve the G-protein signaling, and the CCR5-Env interaction contributes to Env-induced depletion of CD4 T cells, which has been identified by using an Env-mutant R3A recently [6, 16, 18].

In membrane fusion, after Env binding to CD4, gp120 exposes a CD4 induced site (CD4i) which allows the protrusion of one of the V3 loops, both of them will interact with the co-receptors. The V3 loop is the major determinant of R5- and X4-tropism (Fig. **1**). Meanwhile, a hinge region between globular domains 2 and 3 on CD4 bends to move the Env trimer to approach CCR5 and then gp41 undergoes a radical rearrangement and forms a hydrophobic coiled-coil or six-helix bundle that drives fusion between the viral envelope and cell membrane [4, 5, 8, 9].

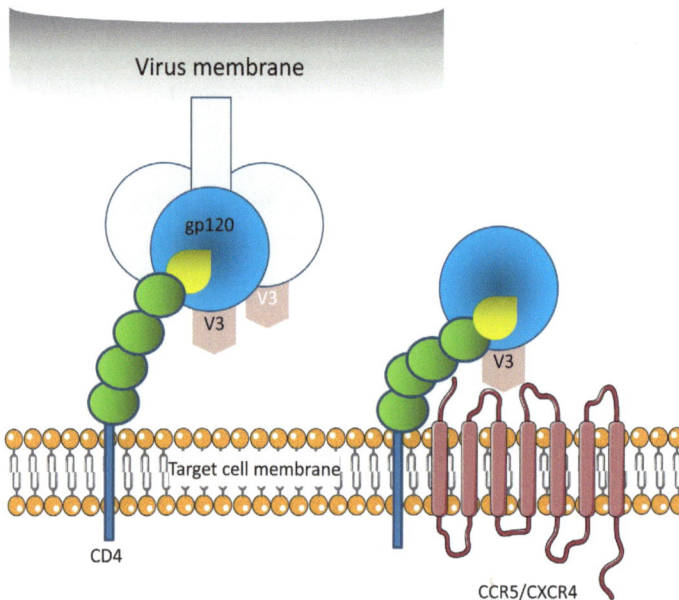

Fig. (1). The interaction between HIV-1 and target cell receptors at the cell surface.

In the past decades, an increasing body of evidence has been provided to unveil the roles of co-receptors signaling in HIV-1 infection. The chemokine receptors, CCR5 and CXCR4, GPCR family members use the G protein-based signal transductions to complete HIV-1 life cycle (Fig. **2**). The chemokine co-receptors bind extracellular ligands, HIV-1 virons or envelope glycoprotein gp120 and induce signal cascades mediated by intracellular plasma membrane-bound heterotrimeric G proteins, thus activating signal pathways influence multi-aspects, including ion flux, cell adhesion, chemotaxis, transcription, cell survival, actin cytoskeleton and microtubule [19]. HIV-1 or its glycoprotein gp120 binding to chemokine co-receptor results in the exchange of G protein complex (a subunit of constitutive heterodimer of β and γ and an α subunit) binding to GTP (guanosine 5'-triphospate) for GDP (guanosine 5'-diphospate), which elicits the dissociation of the βγ heterodimer subunit from the α subunit, and initiates downstream signaling events from all subunits. For instance, Pyk2 (protein tyrosine kinase), PI3K (phosphatidylinositol 3-kinase), threonine kinase Akt, ERK-1/2 (extra-cellular signal-related kinase 1/2) and NFAT (nuclear factor of activated T cells) can be triggered after CXCR4 or CCR5 binding to gp120, and Pyk2 exerts phosphorylation to facilitate cell adhesion which is helpful for viral transmission [19 - 22]. In the previous study, there were sporadic findings implying that co-receptors signaling possibly involved some post-entry steps or viral replication. For instance, CC-chemokines pre-stimulated macrophages or CD4 T cells can enhance HIV-1 replication and some hypotheses explained that co-receptors signaling can influence the viral replication in later steps. Furthermore, it has been found that chemokine receptor signaling can promote HIV-1 to infect the resting CD4 T cells [19, 23 - 27]. Therefore, we cannot deny the important effect of co-receptors signaling in viral infection and the role of co-receptors signaling still has to be studied in the future.

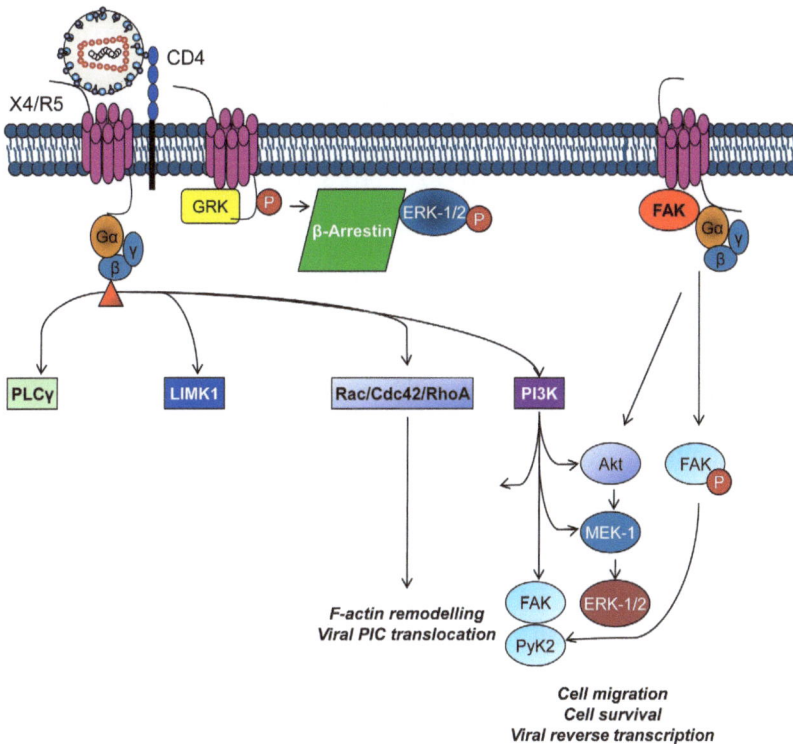

Fig. (2). Signaling pathways involved in HIV and receptors. β-Arr: β -arrestin; GRK: G-protein receptor kinase; PLC-γ: phospholipase C- γ; LIMK1: LIM domain kinase 1; PIC: pre-integration complex; Rac: Ras-related C3 botulinum toxin substrate; Cdc42: Cell division control protein 42 homolog; RhoA: Ras homolog gene family, member A; PI3K: Phosphatidylinositol-4,5-bisphosphate 3-kinase; FAK: focal adhesion kinase; PyK2: proline-rich tyrosine kinase 2; Akt: AKR thymosa 8 provirus homolog; MEK-1: MAPK/ERK kinase 1; ERK-1/2: extracellular regulated protein kinase 1/2.

The HIV-1 Env could simulate the signaling activity of intrinsic chemokines through CCR5 or CXCR4 receptor and G proteins, and to activate various intracellular signaling cascades. It has been shown that high viral antigen levels cause an inappropriate chemotactic host lymphocyte response that can promote viral spread, and co-receptor-mediated signaling pathways may directly influence intracellular steps of the HIV-1 lifecycle [28]. In macrophages, CCR5-mediated G protein signaling pathways play a critical role in HIV-1 replication. Pretreatment of CCR5 ligands promotes HIV-1 infection in a pertussis toxin (PTX)-dependent manner in primary monocytes or monocyte-derived macrophages, suggesting that G protein-mediated signals facilitate a cellular conditions that is highly beneficial to HIV-1 replication [25]. Although it remains unclear whether gp120-induced Pyk2 phosphorylation is Gαi sensitive as observed in cell lines or independent studies in primary macrophages [21, 29], it was clear that the Gαi-Pyk2 activation could elicit MAPK-involved cell survival pathways that allow HIV-1 to replicate in HL60 cell lines [21]. A peptide does not block ligand-receptor interactions was shown to specifically block G protein-mediated chemotaxis pathways [30, 31] and block R5-tropic HIV-1 replication in THP-1 cells, but not X4-tropic viral infection of Jurkat T cells [32]. The detailed mechanism of this specific restriction was not clear, but it appears to occur post-entry, which suggests that CCR5-activated Gαi signaling cascades and downstream events may play a critical role in promoting R5-tropic virus replication in target cells. Later studies have contributed potential mechanisms to illustrate these observations. Paruch and colleagues show that macrophage inflammatiory protein 1 β (MIP-1β) or HIV-1 gp120 binding to CCR5 results in activation of ERK-1/2 and phospholipase D (PLD) signal pathways, which promotes transactivation of the HIV Tat and LTR by NF-κB transcription factor *in vitro* [33]. Further experiment demonstrated that knockdown of either PLD1 or PLD2 substantially inhibits HIV infection in THP-1 monocytic cells. Although the overall inhibition of HIV-1 replication could be observed by abrogation of Gαi signaling, the specific G protein activation-dependent PLD pathway activation was not shown. More studies have shown that HIV-1 gp120 can also induce activation of Ca^{2+} release in a PTX-sensitive manner in primary activated T cells and macrophages, as well as the activation of PI3K and Akt signalings (Fig. **2**) [34]. This activity is deemed to eliminate a block to HIV-1 replication at a liable point after viral reverse transcription but before integration, which again implies the critical role for G protein signaling in facilitating CCR5-mediated viral replication in macrophages.

There is evidence that in CD4[+] T cells, high density of CCR5 at the cell surface correlates with an increased level of HIV-1 replication, which suggests a similar role of G protein signaling for CCR5. It was observed that a 2-fold increase in viral particles entering the cytosol of cells expressing high level CCR5 results in a 30- to 80-fold increase in overall viral replication at the stage after reverse transcription but before integration step. This increase is blocked by the treatment of PTX, which implies the replication increase is associated with G protein signaling [35]. These observations were further proved by study in primary T-cells expressing CCR5 mutants that is incapable of signaling through Gαi proteins thus poorly supported HIV-1 replication [36]. In these results, non-activated T-cells were employed to prevent excessive cellular activation from belying the role of these signaling pathways. Furthermore, it has been shown that the overexpression of wild-type CCR5 co-receptor in the human osteoblast (HOS) cell line and in primary peripheral blood mononucleated cell (PBMC) increases HIV-1 replication, while the overexpression of signaling-defective mutants does not. Both PTX-treatment and Gαi-specific siRNA knockdown experiments suggest that this is due to lack of Gαi-associated signals, although it is unknown which stage of the viral lifecycle is authentically affected [37]. This work suggests that not only the requirement of Gαi signals for the HIV-1 lifecycle, but also the activation state of primary cells or transformed cell lines may be strongly associated with the outcome of experiments aimed to assess the role of G protein signaling in viral replication. The further data demonstrate that MAPK pathway activation by gp120 in the context of T cell receptor (TCR) stimulation but not IL-7 stimulation, which supports the aforementioned idea [38]. Additional evidence show that the treatment of primary cells with RANTES facilitates X4-tropic HIV replication in a Gαi-dependent manner, but does not increase the CXCR4 expression on cell surface, which suggests that CCR5 signaling may be important at the post-viral entry stages [23]. In contrast, however, there is one study suggests that Gαi-mediated beta chemokine signaling decreases cyclic adenosine monophosphate (cAMP) and PKA activation, bywhich inhibits HIV replication in primary lymphocytes, an observation needed to be tested further [39]. A solid investigation shows that both R5- and X4-tropic viruses are capable of inducing MAPK/ERKsignal pathway activation but not p38/JNK activation in unstimulated PBMC, which contributes the compelling mechanistic evidence for the role of CCR5 or CXCR4 Gαi signals in post-entry viral replication [40]. It demonstrated that the ERK activation is dependent on Gαi signals, and the ERK-activation is required for the late stages of HIV-1 reverse transcription. This study challenges the previous suggestions that R5-tropic virus can activate MAPK/ERK and p38/JNK signal pathways [41] but the ERK pathway does not affect R5 viral replication [42], and that X4-tropic virus is unable to activate the MAPK/ERK pathway [43]. These discrepancies may be due, in part, to the use of less suitable cells lines such as Jurkat cell line and SIV-infection models in older studies.

Like the R5-tropic virus requires G protein and associated signalings for viral replication, increasing evidence supports the idea that X4-tropic strains have similar requirements as well. The addition of the CXCR4 ligand SDF-1α to HIV-infected Jurkat cells activates ERK in a Gαi-dependent manner and enhances viral replication, which is in consistence with the data observed in the CCR5 signaling case [44]. Pre-incubation of cells with PTX also potentially inhibits X4-tropic viral strain infection in primary PBMC [45]. In primary T cells, PTX pre-treatment abrogates soluble gp120-elicited Tat-Sf1 expression, which implicates that CXCR4-mediated G protein signals are able to facilitate the stimulation of HIV LTR [46]. Recently, CXCR4-mediated Gαi signals have been shown to be able to overcome the actin-based restriction of HIV infection in resting T cells [27]. The Gαi pathways activate cofilin and elicit actin depolymerization, thus allowing the viral pre-integration complex (PIC) enter nuclear. Block of this pathway strongly abrogates latent infection in resting T cells, which indicates an important role for G protein signaling during HIV latent infection in T cells. Taken together, these studies suggest that in both macrophages and T cells, through either CCR5 or CXCR4, G protein signalings play a crucial role in facilitating HIV replication at multiple steps during the viral replication cycle. These studies shed new light on the potential of molecules involved in signaling complex for HIV-1 therapy. Attempts to design small molecule compound or endogenous analogues or effective antibodies to impact the chemokine co-receptor-induced signaling pathways or co-receptors function are underway in different laboratories.

II. ANTAGONIST-BASED ON DIFFERENT MECHANISMS

In recent decades, an increasing number of investigations have focused on chemokine receptor-based HIV-1 entry inhibitors. Enormous progress has been made, especially for CCR5-based antagonists which include an in the market and a pro-list monoclonal antibody (mAb) drug. Here are some typical delegates of inhibitors depend on different regulatory mechanisms of co-receptors in viral entry.

ANTAGONISTS BASED ON-CCR5

The Biology of CCR5

CCR5 is predominantly expressed on the surface of a number of cell types, including activated or memory CD4$^+$ and CD8$^+$ T cells, macrophages, natural killer (NK) cells, NKT cells, eosinophils, microglia and astrocytes. CCR5 consists of an N-terminal extracellular tail, seven transmembrane α-helices which are linked by three intracellular loops (ICL1-3), three extracellular loops (ECL1-3), and a C-terminal cytoplasmic tail (Fig. **3**) [47]. The N-terminal domain and the ECLs are required for Env-mediated fusion [48], the Aspartic acid 11, Lysine 197 and Aspartic acid 276 in the two functional regions contribute to the Env-cell membrane fusion. ECL2 forms a β-hairpin structure and interact with V3 loop of HIV-1 gp120 in the viral entry process, which can motivate virus-host cell membrane fusion [49]. Besides, both ECL2 and N-terminal region are major binding determinants for CCR5 ligands [50], that is why more and more HIV-1 researchers pay much attention to CCR5 antagonists. Firstly, CCR5 was identified as a functional GPCR that is antagonized by three CC chemokines, which include MIP-1α (CCL3), MIP-1β (CCL4) and RANTES (Regulated upon Activation, Normal T cell Expressed and presumably Secreted, CCL5) [51, 52]. It was later found that several other CC chemokines, monocyte chemotactic proteins (MCP-1, MCP-2, MCP-3 and MCP-4) and eotaxin, can bind CCR5 with different affinities and efficiencies in receptor activation [53]. Up to now, there are eight chemokines have been identified as CCR5 ligands (Table **1**).

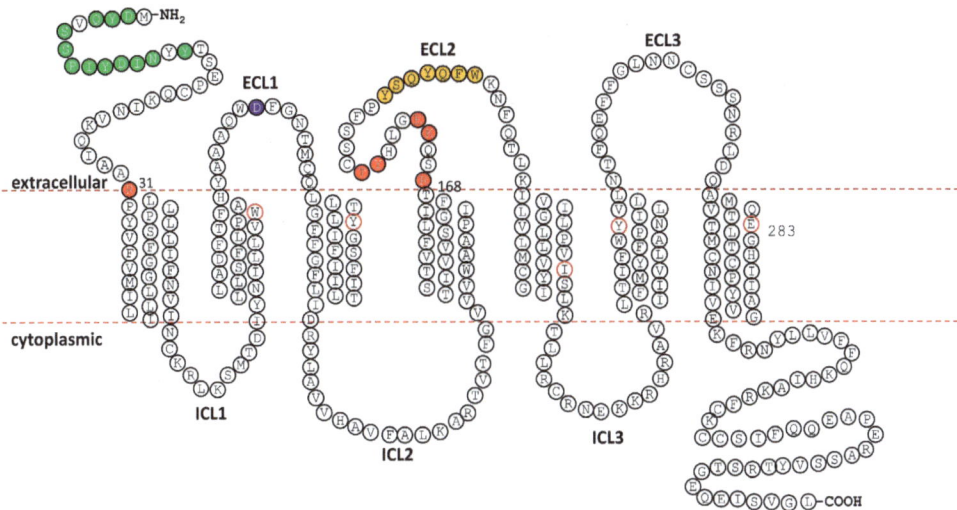

Fig. (3). The schematic structure of human CCR5.

Table 1. Chemokines and chemokine receptors associated with CCR5.

Chemokines		Chemokine Receptors
Systemic Name	**Common Name**	
CCL2	MCP-1	CCR2, CCR4
CCL3	MIP-1α	CCR1, CCR4, CCR5
CCL4	MIP-1β	CCR5
CCL5	RANTES	CCR1, CCR3, CCR5
CCL7	MCP-3	CCR1, CCR2, CCR3, CCR5
CCL8	MCP-2	CCR1, CCR2B, CCR3, CCR5
CCL13	MCP-4	CCR2, CCR3, CCR5
CCL3L1	LD78β	CCBP2, CCR5

MCP-3, also called CCL7, is a natural antagonist for CCR5. MIP-1α, MIP-1β and RANTES are HIV-suppressive factors produced by CD8$^+$ T cells, which can induce CCR5 endocytosis and contribute to the control of HIV infection *in vivo* [5, 53, 54]. MIP-1α, MIP-1β, and RANTES are full agonists that bind efficiently to CCR5, whereas MCP-3, CCL8 (MCP-2), and MCP-4 (CCL13) bind less efficiently and reveal different capacities in receptor activation. Intriguingly, MCP-3 has been found to bind CCR5 without activating a signal, and it could also inhibit the activation of CCR5 by MIP-1β [53]. Among the several CC chemokines bind CCR5, MIP-1α, MIP-1β, RANTES, and MCP-2 demonstrate the strongest activities in suppressing HIV-1 infection [53]. MCP-3 binds efficiently to CCR5, but does not induce the co-receptor internalization or block HIV-1 infection [53]. Interestingly, MCP-1 binds to CCR5 and acts as a potential enhancer rather than a blocker of HIV-1 replication [55]. CCL3L1 (Chemokine C-C motif ligand 3-like 1) is also called LD78β, it binds to CCR5 and inhibits HIV entry [56]. Therefore, it is rational to produce these CCR5 ligands or their functional analogs and utilize them to inhibit the function of CCR5 to treat and prevent AIDS. Furthermore, CCR5, like most seven transmembrane GPCRs, spans the plasma membrane seven times in a serpentine manner [57]. The CCR5 extracellular combination of the amino-terminal domain (Nt) and the second extracellular loop (ECL2) represents potential targets for HIV-inhibitory mAbs. The sulfation of Nt tyrosines has been shown to promote gp120 binding, thus facilitating HIV-1 entry [58, 59].

CCR5 antagonists

The antagonists of CCR5 are composed of chemokine-derived peptides, non-peptide small molecules, mAbs, and peptide compounds. A series studies of site-directed mutagenesis and molecular modeling of CCR5 have identified a putative binding site in a cavity between the transmembrane helices on the extracellular portion of CCR5 that is shared by several CCR5 small-molecule inhibitors [57, 60 - 64]. Competitive binding site determination studies demonstrate that this site is paetaken by various small-molecule inhibitors of CCR5 [9, 64]. This site is not overlapped with the binding site for HIV gp120, which is located on the extracellular domains of CCR5 [63]. The entry inhibitors currently in clinical trials based-on CCR5 co-receptor are shown in Table **2**. The suffix '-viroc' which comes from the initials of viral receptor occupancy has been assigned as generic names for the mall-molecule antagonists based on CCR5The tested "-viroc" antagonists exhibit potent inhibition of all clades of group M HIV-1, including laboratory-adapted and primary isolated strains, replication *in vitro* . Meanwhile, these agents do not possess agonist properties and do not affect the expression level of CCR5 at cell surface. In addition, the CCR5 mAbs have displayed broad and potent anti-HIV-1 activity *in vitro* [65]. Clinical studies have established

CCR5 mAbs as potent antiretroviral agents with prolonged activity following a single dose. CCR5 mAbs represent both a distinct class of CCR5 inhibitor and a novel approach to HIV-1 therapy.

Table 2. CCR5 inhibitors that have been clinically testing as HIV therapeutics.

Molecule	Class	Status	Comments
Cenicriviroc	Small molecule	Phase IIb	
INCB-9471	Small molecule	Phase II	some mild side effects
Maraviroc	Small molecule	Oral Maraviroc for use as HIV pre-exposure prophylaxis (PrEP) is in Phase II development. Topical microbicide formulations of Maraviroc are in Phase I development.	
Monomeric DAPTA	peptides	Phase II	no significant clinical side effects
Vicriviroc	Small molecule	Vicriviroc-containing microbicides for HIV prevention are in Phase I studies.	
PRO140	mAb	Phase IIb/III	

a). Maraviroc

A 32-base-pair deletion in the CCR5 gene (CCR5Δ32) was found to be responsible for a non-functional CCR5 that prevents membrane fusion and hence interdicts R5-tropic strains from entering target cells [66, 67]. This discovery brings new inspiration to HIV investigators, who have tried many strategies to mimic the function of CCR5Δ32/CCR5Δ32 phenotype. Maraviroc is a successful example, which was selected from nearly 1 000 analogues of a small-molecule CCR5 ligand named imidazopyridine UK-107 543 (Fig. **4**). Maraviroc is a selective CCR5 antagonist with a half maximal inhibitory concentration (IC_{50}) of 6.4 nM, it displays potent anti-HIV-1 activity by preventing the interaction of HIV-1 gp120 and CCR5 and inhibiting HIV-1 entry. Maraviroc is the first and only CCR5 antagonist and has been approved for use in HIV-1 treatment in 2007. Maraviroc functions *via* a new allosteric mechanism different from other approved antiretroviral drugs, which can restrain the downstream CCR5 signaling after interacting with cognate chemokine, and compete with the soluble subunit of gp120 to bind to a hydrophobic pocket on CCR5 to prevent the membrane fusion, without altering CCR5 cell surface levels and CCR5-associated intracellular signaling. Maraviroc also can inhibit MIP-1α, MIP-1β, and RANTES binding to CCR5, intracellular calcium influx induced by chemokine, and chemokine-dependent GDP-GTP exchange. Therefore, Maraviroc provides robust protection against all R5-tropic HIV-1 viruses [12, 61, 68, 69].

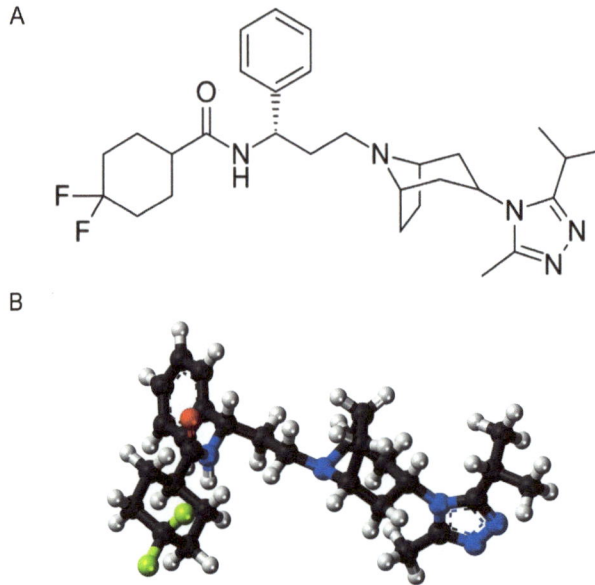

Fig. (4). The chemical structure of Maraviroc.

In phase 1 clinical trials, single-dose intravenous (i.v.) and oral administration (p.o.) of Maraviroc to both male Sprague-Dawley (SD) rats and male beagle dogs were used to predicted pharmacokinetic values. The experimental results showed that clearance values and half-life values in rat species were 74 ml/min/kg and 0.9 h respectively, in dog species were 21 ml/min/kg and 2.3 h respectively. The volume of distribution in both species were 4.3 to 6.5 liters/kg (1 mg/kg i.v for rats, 0.5 mg/kg i.v. for dogs). These data were used to allometric scaling to humans which proofed that the dose of exposure above the geometric mean antiviral IC90 was 100 mg twice a day (BID), and the dose of 25 mg once daily (QD) was close to maximum saturation level [12, 70].

The phase 2 clinical trials estimated the effect of Maraviroc monotherapy in viral load compared with placebo, and assessed its safety and tolerability. A total of 82 patients were divided into eight groups to receive Maraviroc treatment of 25 mg, 100 mg, 300 mg QD and 50 mg, 100 mg, 150 mg (fed and fasted), 300 mg BID and other two groups to receive placebo treatment. After a short-term monotherapy of Maraviroc and placebo, eight Maraviroc treatment groups had a larger decrease in viral load than placebo groups, except one patient treated with 100 mg BID showing no declined in viral load. The clinical trials results indicated that Maraviroc was well-tolerated at doses from 25 mg to 300 mg. The doses of ≥100 mg BID resulted in average maximum HIV-1 RNA reductions exceed 1.5log10 [71]. In later tropism analysis, the X4-tropic virus appeared in two patients at 11 days, but it was not detectable in the other sixty patients. These data indicated that X4-tropic virus do not emerge rapidly *in vivo* after receiving Maraviroc therapy [72]. Finally, phase 3 clinical trials assessed the efficacy and safety of Maraviroc, which includes 48 weeks double-blind treatment, open-label Maraviroc twice daily treatment between 48-week and 96-week and five years safety evaluation of Maraviroc. Efficacy analysis showed the average decrease in HIV-1 RNA levels and increase in CD4 cell count with Maraviroc once daily and twice daily therapy were better than the placebo group. Safety analysis showed Maraviroc caused adverse events like diarrhea, fatigue, fever, headache, nausea and rash which are similar to placebo, whereas upper respiratory tract infection caused by Maraviroc was more serious than placebo. In addition, 5 percent patients were found with different forms of cancer thus result in death in five years safety evaluation of Maraviroc [73 - 75].

To sum up, Maraviroc has a greater ability of inhibiting viruses and increasing CD4 T cells than placebo, and is safe and well tolerated compared with other drugs despite of some adverse events. These significant studies led to FDA approval. It's noteworthy that Maraviroc antagonist only inhibits R5-tropic HIV, and may impel viruses to use CXCR4 under the selection pressure and result in CD4 cell decline [11, 76]. Therefore, we should pay more attention on the appearance of X4-tropic and the side effect during MAC therapy or use combination drug therapy to control R5-tropic and X4-tropic simultaneously. Besides, we can modify the structure of Maraviroc in order to prolong half-life, increase patients' compliance and reduce adverse events. Maraviroc is currently a good choice to treat HIV-infected patients with R5-tropic virus before we find another safer, more effective and broad-spectrum drug to replace it.

b). Cenicrivivoc

The side effects and inefficiency of the first-generation "viroc" agents based on-CCR5, prompted development of next-genenration CCR5 antagonists. Cenicriviroc is a most promising one in the clinical pipelines [77]. Cenicriviroc, also called TAK-652, is a derivative of the first small-molecular nonpeptide CCR5 co-receptor antagonist TAK-779. It prevents viral entry by binding to a domain of CCR5 which blocking the interaction between HIV-1 gp120 and CCR5 (Fig. **5**) [78, 79]. Cenicriviroc is also a dual chemokine receptor (CCR5/CCR2) antagonist [80], it inhibits the binding of MIP-1α, MIP-1β and RANTES to CCR5-expressing cells at nanomolar concentrations [78], and could also suppress the binding of MCP-1 to CCR2b-expressing cells. Cenicriviroc has been studied for the treatment of HIV infection and is being studied for the treatment of HIV-associated neurocognitive disease (HAND) [80]. It is also being studied for inflammatory and fibrotic conditions, including non-alcoholic steatohepatitis

(NASH) and primary sclerosing cholangitis (PSC) [81, 82]. Cenicriviroc has a long plasma half-life of 30 to 40 hours and requires only once-daily dosing [83]. In a study of a Cenicriviroc-resistant clinical isolate, it was shown that simultaneous several amino acid changes in the V3 region and the other Env regions were required for the complete resistance to Cenicriviroc by R5-tropic HIV-1 [84]. Intriguingly, Cenicriviroc demonstrated strong inhibition of the replication of some strains with multidrug-resistance to NRTIs, NNRTIs, and PIs. The working concentrations are similar to those that suppressing the replication of isolated strain from treatment-naïve patient [78].

Fig. (5). The chemical structure of Cenicriviroc.

In a Phase I/II 10-day monotherapy dose-escalating study (clinical trial No. NCT01092104), which included treatment-experienced and CCR5-antagonis--naive HIV-infected patients, there was only one shift in viral tropism was observed. Accordingly, the one participant demonstrated a tropism shift from CCR5 to CXCR4 co-receptor at baseline was excluded from later efficacy analysis [80]. In a 48-week Phase IIb study (NCT01338883), 143 treatment-naive HIV-infected participants received either once-daily Cenicriviroc (115 patients, 100 mg or 200 mg) or once-daily Efavirenz (28 patients), each in combination with Emtricitabine/Tenofovir DF (Truvada). In this study, virologic failure (VF) occurred in 10 out of 115 (8.7%) Cenicriviroc-treated participants and in 1 out of 28 (3.6%) Efavirenz-treated participants. In addition, 5 Cenicriviroc-treated participants had NRTI resistance mutations (M184I and/or V) and demonstrated VF. However, 4 of the 5 participants had suboptimal Cenicriviroc plasma concentrations. The NRTI mutations accounted for 75% of the 100 mg Cenicriviroc VFs and for 33% of the 200 mg Cenicriviroc VFs. In contrast, none of the Efavirenz-treated participants with VF had emergent NRTI mutations. One participant occurred VF in the 200-mg Cenicriviroc group experienced a tropism switch from CCR5 to D/M-tropic virus [85].

c). INCB-9471

INCB-9471 is a small-molecule CCR5 co-receptor antagonist that selectively and reversibly binds to a CCR5 binding pocket that is different to which maraviroc binds (Fig. **6**). INCB-9471 blocks viral entry by inhibiting the interaction between HIV-1 gp120 and CCR5. The prevention of INCB-9471 on CCR5-mediated viral entry is through allosteric noncompetitive mechanisms. INCB-9471 does not inhibit CXCR4-tropic or dual-tropic viruses [86, 87]. The half-life of INCB-9471 is approximately 60 hours, and it is eliminated primarily by CYP3A-mediated metabolism.

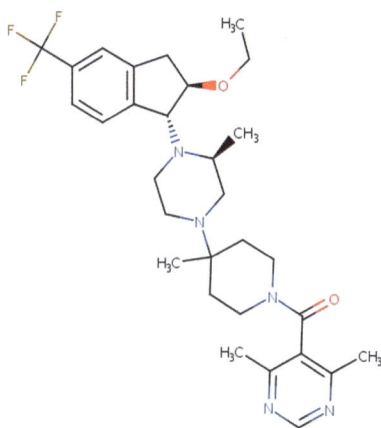

Fig. (6). The chemical structure of INCB-9471.

In a 14-day monotherapy study of 200 mg INCB-9471, the R5-tropic HIV-infected, treatment-naive and -experienced adults were included. The result demonstrated that 2 treatment-experienced participants out of 19 INCB-947--treated participants (10.5%) showed a tropism change from R5 to D/M-tropic virus [88]. Preliminary analysis suggested that the X4-using viruses in D/M tropic-viruses derived from the pre-existing viral variants. In both participants, virus reverted back to R5-tropic 28 days after therapy.

In a separate 14-day monotherapy study (designated as INCB 9471-201), the once-daily dose of 100, 200, or 300 mg INCB-9471 was given to R5-tropic HIV-infected adults respectively. The result showed that D/M tropic virus emerged in 4 participants, two participants in the 200 mg group and two participants in the 300 mg group, out of 39 who completed INCB-9471 treatment. Analysis on the two participants receiving the once-daily 200 mg dose of INCB-9471 suggested that emergence of X4-using viral variants reflected outgrowth from pre-treatment viral reservoirs [89].

d). Monomeric DAPTA (mDAPTA)

mDAPTA is a reformulated monomeric form of a synthetic octapeptide compound called peptide T ([D-Ala$_1$] peptide T amide; DAPTA), it derived from the HIV gp120 V2 region (Fig. **7**). Peptide T is a selective CCR5 co-receptor antagonist directly binds to the CCR5 co-receptor. Tt prevents viral entry by inhibiting the interaction between HIV-1 gp120 and CCR5 [90 - 92]. It has been shown that mDAPTA is able to inhibit the release of X4- and R5-tropic HIV from CD8-depleted PBMCs isolated from HIV-negative patients and HIV-positive patients with viral load below 50 copies/mL *in vitro*. mDAPTA has also been studied for its antiviral effect on the human polyomavirus JC strain. In individuals with progressive multifocal leukoencephalopathy (PML), an anti-viral effect of mDAPTA was observed. In a Phase I study of mDAPTA plasma kinetics, the participants with AIDS or AIDS-related complex (ARC) following intravenous (IV) or intranasal (IN) administration were involved. The data demonstrated that mDAPTA had a biphasic plasma kinetics, which was featured with a first compartment half-life of 30 to 60 minutes and a second plasma clearance time of 4 to 6 hours [93].

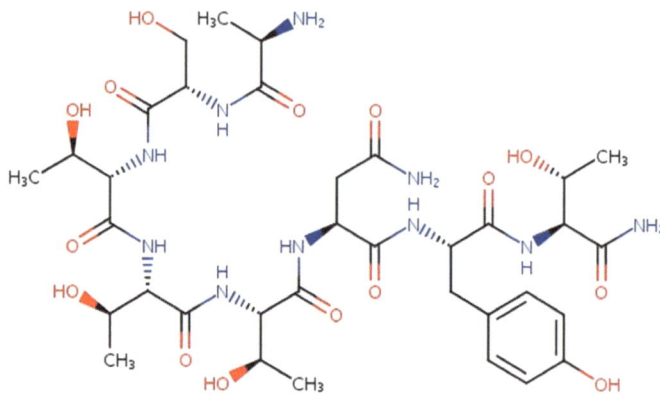

Fig. (7). The chemical structure of mDAPTA.

The data of the Phase I study show that the drug could not be detected in urine in patients with AIDS or ARC after receiving peptide T *via* IV or IN administration [93]. In a small study of 11 HIV-infected participants receiving mDAPTA either alone or in combination with current ART drugs for up to 32 weeks, no obvious CCR5 to CXCR4 co-receptor shift was observed, and there was no treatment-resistant viruses emerged [94].

e). Vicriviroc

Vicriviroc is a reversible, noncompetitive allosteric small-molecule pyrimidine antagonist of CCR5 co-receptor. It binds to a small hydrophobic pocket of the CCR5 extracellular surface, and subsequently induces conformational change of the surface segment, thus inhibiting the binding of HIV-1 gp120 to CCR5 of target cells and prevents viral entry (Fig. **8**) [86, 95, 96]. The half-life of Vicriviroc is 28 hours in HIV-infected individuals treated by 50 mg of oral Vicriviroc twice daily [86]. Vicriviroc is primarily metabolized by CYP3A4, and by CYP3A5 and CYP2C9 to a lesser extent [86]. In a metabolism study with healthy participants received a single ^{14}C-radiolabeled dose of Vicriviroc, the data indicated that approximately 47% of Vicriviroc was excreted in urine, and 45% of Vicriviroc was excreted in feces [97].

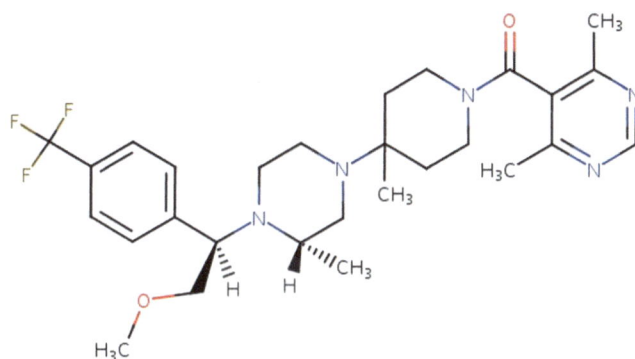

Fig. (8). The chemical structure of Vicriviroc.

In two Phase III trials of oral Vicriviroc, the viruses from treatment-experienced participants experiencing VF were isolated and analyzed. Only those participants with R5-tropic virus detected at baseline were included for analysis. There were 71 out of 486 Vicriviroc-treated participants met the protocol-defined VF criteria after 48 weeks of treatment. Of those virologic failures, 10% were determined to have D-M/X4 viral strains at the time of failure. Four out of 486 (1%) treated participants was identified as resistance to Vicriviroc (). Clonal analysis demonstrated that 2 to 5 amino acid substitutions in the V3 loop are associated with Vicriviroc resistance. Although the changes outside the V3 loop were observed in resistant clones, no consistent pattern was found [98]. Further *in vitro* studies showed that the weakened susceptibility to Vicriviroc is associated with mutations in the gp120 V4 loop and the gp41 fusion peptide of HIV-1 [99, 100].

f). PRO140

PRO140 is a humanized CCR5 monoclonal antibody that binds to CCR5 and has potent antiretroviral activity in individuals infected with R5-tropic rather than inhibiting X4-tropic. It is a competitive inhibitorof HIV-1 entry and transmission which comprises binding to CCR5 extracellular epitopes include D2 domain of the amino terminus and R168 in ECL2, blocking gp120-CD4 binding and calcium fluxes and inhibiting cell membrane fusion [101, 102]. PRO140 and small molecule CCR5 antagonists synergize with a natural ligand for CCR5, RANTES. Both of them shows potent antiviral synergy when they are combined, but PRO140 does not block CCR5 natural function *in vitro* which is quite different from small molecule CCR5 antagonists [102, 103]. In previous years, some research groups designed phase 1 clinical trials to assess the anti-HIV activity, safety, and pharmacokinetics of i.v. PRO 140 single-dose of 0.5 mg/kg, 2 mg/kg, 5 mg/kg. Compared with the placebo group, PRO140 had a better antiviral effect. It was identified that HIV-1 RNA load reduced at least $1.0\log_{10}$ copies/mL after PRO140 treatment and the anti-HIV response rate of 5 mg/kg was 100 percent. Some adverse events appeared after patients were treated with PRO140 and placebo, 31% patients had a headache, 28% patients had lymphadenopathy, and both diarrhea and fatigue were 21%. The pharmacokinetics date of 0.5 mg/kg, 2 mg/kg, and 5 mg/kg PRO140 i.v. showed mean half-life of 1.5 days, 3.5 days and 3.9 days respectively, and the average PRO140 peak concentration was 13 g/mL, 61 g/mL, and 173 g/mL respectively. These experimental data proved that use 5 mg/kg as PRO140 single-dose can produce potent and prolonged antiviral activity and increase CD4 cell count [103].

In phase 2 clinical trials, virological evaluations, bioanalytical methods, pharmacokinetic and pharmacodynamic analyses were used to assess therapeutic effect through subcutaneous injection of PRO140 162 mg weekly, 324mg weekly, 324mg biweekly for two doses and intravenous injection single dose of 5mg/kg and 10mg/kg. The mean HIV-1 RNA reduction of PRO140 162 mg weekly, 324 mg weekly, 324 mg biweekly, 5 mg/kg dose, 10 mg/kg dose, and placebo were $0.99\log_{10}$, $1.65\log_{10}$, $1.37\log_{10}$, $1.84\log_{10}$, $2.09\log_{10}$ and $0.23\log_{10}$ respectively, these data proved PRO140 has a better anti-HIV effect relative to placebo. Only a few subjects had diarrhea, headache, nasal congestion, lymphadenopathy, and hypertension during PRO140 therapeutic process. It is noteworthy that anti-PRO140 antibodies were detected in all PRO140 groups though it had a little effect on the pharmacokinetics or viral load reductions. The detection results demonstrated that PRO140 *via* subcutaneous injection presents the potential for HIV-1 replication suppression and rare patient self-administration, 5 mg/kg or 10 mg/kg single-dose intravenous infusion exhibits potent, prolonged antiretroviral activity and good tolerance [13, 14]. At present, PRO140 are not approved for HIV-1 therapy, but all research listed above has proofed the idea that PRO140 indeed have application prospect in AIDS treatment. In addition, more clinical trials are required to identify whether the appearance of anti-PRO 140 antibodies will decline the antiviral efficacy of PRO140 in long-term therapy or not.

ANTAGONISTS BASED ON-CXCR4

The Biology of CXCR4

CXCR4, also called leukocyte-derived seven-transmembrane domain receptor (LESTR), was originally identified as an orphan receptor in early 1990s (Fig. **9**) [104 - 108]. It did not receive much attention until its isolation as an indispensable co-receptor (called fusin) for HIV-1 infection in T lymphocytes [16] and the discovery of its natural ligand, SDF-1/CXCL12 [109, 110]. The identification of CXCR4 as an HIV co-receptor [16] brought a large number of research activities to investigate the biological roles of the CXCL12/CXCR4 axis in HIV-1 replication. CXCL12 is a highly conserved chemokine in mammals. The CCL12 of mouse and human shares 99% homology, which allows it to act across species barriers. Recently, there are a total of six isoforms have been identified for the CXCL12 [111]. It was shown that CXCL12g is a very weak agonist for CXCR4, but it is at least 5-6 times more potent than CXCL12a in HIV-blocking assays [112]. The potent blocking activity of CXCL12g to HIV-1 is strongly dependent on its activity to induce efficient CXCR4 internalization in target cells.

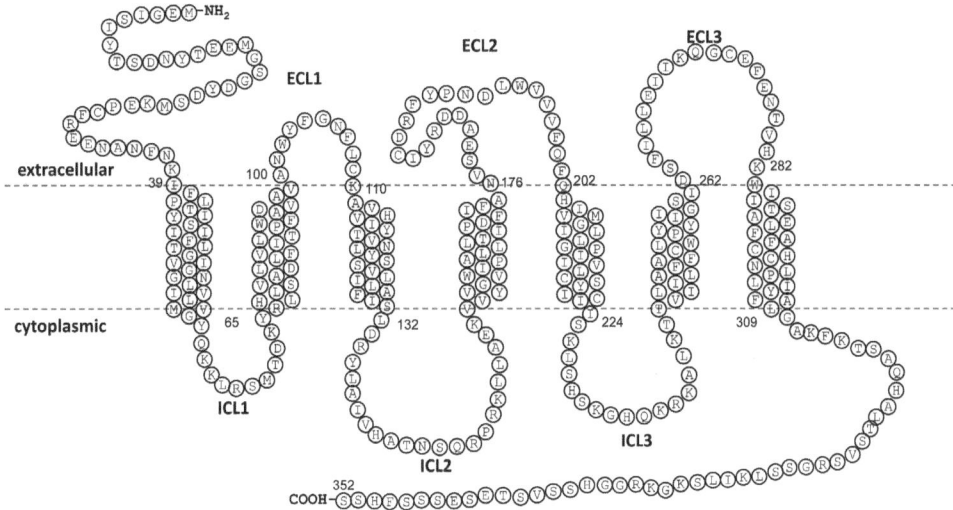

Fig. (9). Schematic structure of CXCR4.

CXCR4 Antagonists

AMD3100

Compared to CCR5 antagonists, few works have been done in order to investigate CXCR4 antagonists for treating HIV-1 infections. However, as we know, many

HIV-1infected patients carry both R5-tropic and X4-tropic, and the X4-tropic may become predominant under the selection pressure with the disease progresses [6, 76]. Thus, it is an urgent task for us to develop novel CXCR4 inhibitors, which would increase the possibility to treat patients infected with X4-tropic or dual-tropic X4/R5 HIV-1 strains. AMD3100, a CXCR4 antagonist, can inhibit the infection of X4-tropic selectively, but was found that have the capability of mobilizing hematopoietic stem and progenitor cells simultaneously (Fig. **10**) [113, 114]. CX6, a CXCR4 small molecule inhibitor, utilizes the hydrogen bond interactions with Asp97 and Glu288 to bind CXCR4. CX6 inhibits the fusion between HIV-1NL4-3 envelope and CXCR4 with IC50 of 1.9 μM, exerts anti-HIV-1 activity with IC50 of 1.5 μM, blocks the SDF-1α induced intracellular Ca^{2+} mobilization with IC50 of 92 nM [115].

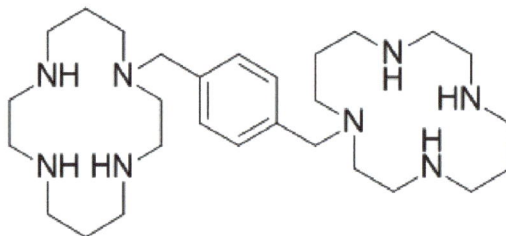

Fig. (10). Structure of AMD3100.

AMD-070

AMD-070 is a selective and reversible small molecule antagonist for chemokine co-receptor CXCR4 (Fig. **11**) [116]. AMD-070 binds to transmembrane regions of CXCR4, and blocking the interaction of the CD4–gp120 complex with the ECL2 domain of the CXCR4 co-receptor, thus prevents CXCR4-mediated viral entry of T-cell tropic synctium-inducing HIV-1, which is associated with advanced stages of HIV-1 infection [116].

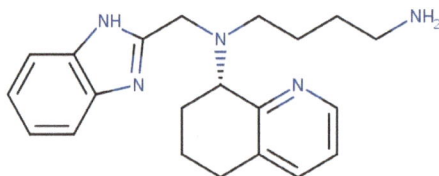

Fig. (11). Structure of AMD-070.

In healthy participants, the median estimated terminal half-life of AMD-070 ranged from 7.6 to 12.6 hours in single-dose cohorts administrated with 50 mg to

400 mg, and from 11.2 to 15.9 hours in multiple-dose cohorts administrated with 100 mg to 400 mg twice daily [117]. AMD-070 is primarily eliminated by metabolism, with less than 1% of the oral administration dose appearing unchanged in the urine. The *in vitro* studies using human liver microsomes have demonstrated that AMD-070 is metabolized by CYP3A4 and by CYP2D6 to a lesser extent [116]. AMD-070 is a substrate of P-glycoprotein (P-gp) [116]. In a 10-day monotherapy study designated XACT, 100 mg or 200 mg of AMD-070 twice daily was administrated in 10 HIV-infected adults. Among them, nine participants had D/M-tropic virus and one had X4-tropic virus were determined by screening with Trofile assay . One participant was determined to be non-evaluable. Of four responders achieving a reduction in X4-tropic virus population of greater than or equal to 1 log10 relative luminescence units (RLU), three participants demonstrated a shift from D/M-tropic virus to R5-tropic virus. The shift to R5 tropism reverted back to D/M tropism following completion of treatment by Day 30. Of the non-responders, all but one participant maintained tropism during the whole therapy period, with the latter participant showing a shift from X4 tropism to D/M tropism on Day 5, which reverted back to X4 by Day 17 [118]. In another 10-day monotherapy study (designated ACTG A5210) of twice daily AMD-070 200 mg in six HIV-infected adults, all six studied participants were D/M-tropic at study entry. At Day 10, all participants remained D/M-tropic except for one participant was only R5-tropic virus.

The Phase I/II monotherapy study (clinical trial number NCT0036110110), it aimed to evaluate the safety and antiviral efficiency of AMD-070. The study involved adults with evidence of CXCR4-using (X4- or D-tropic HIV) HIV-infection, the participants were treatment-naive or treatment-experienced (discontinued ART for at least 14 days prior to study entry). The 200 mg of AMD-070 was orally administered twice daily over 10 days. Notably, two patients received 100 mg of AMD-070 twice daily instead of the protocol-defined 200 mg dose by dosing error [118]. This study came to a stop because of liver toxicity seen in animal studies. In the completed NCT0036110110 clinical trial study, a total of six study drug-related adverse events were reported among five participants involved [118]. All except one was reported of drug-related adverse event was of grade I severity. The most common adverse events were mild gastrointestinal symptoms such as diarrhea and flatulence, and some participants displayed headache. Dizziness was also observed in one participant. Neither drug-related serious adverse events nor laboratory abnormalities of grade I or higher were reported. Hepatotoxicity was also not observed during this study [118]. The other phase I/II monotherapy study evaluated the safety and antiviral efficiency of AMD-070 (clinical trial number NCT0008946611) beyond the NCT0036110110 clinical trial was conducted. The evidenced CXCR4-using (X4- or D-tropic HIV) HIV-infected, treatment-naive or -experienced (discontinued ART for at least 14 days prior to study entry) adults were involved. Twice daily oral administration of 200 mg of AMD-070 was conducted for over 10 days. In the NCT0008946611 trail, no adverse events of grade III severity or higher were observed following 7 days therapy or during the whole treatment period. Taken together, the AMD-070 is basically safe for treatment of X4-tropic virus-infected patients.

NOVEL ANTAGONISTS BASED ON CO-RECEPTOR-INTERACTING PROTEINS

The GPCRs complete internalization or desensitization on cell membrane by recruiting intracellular proteins like β-arrestin 1 (Fig. **12**) [119 - 121]. To study the infection mechanism and identify relevant factors can help us find an effective treatment for HIV-1 infection. There is no doubt that Env, CD4 receptor, and chemokine receptors play a significant role in HIV infection. Recently, some co-receptor-interacting proteins were found to be key regulators in CCR5 or CXCR4 expression and internalization, and the expression of these receptors motivate the HIV entry into host cells [122, 123]. β-arrestin 1 regulates the CCR5 post-endocytic sorting in different cell apparatii when stimulated with PSC-RANTES and 5P14-RANTES [124], which implies that the host factors interacting with co-receptors determine their fate and sequential viral replication. Recently, Spear M *et al*. proposed that targeting HIV-dependent host cofactors are novel anti-HIV therapeutics, especially the factors targeting HIV-mediated chemotactic signaling and actin dynamics involved in co-receptors [125]. In combination with others and our work, the molecules involved in the chemokine receptors CCR5 and CXCR4-mediated signal pathways are the novel therapeutic targets for development of anti-viral drugs.

NHERF1

The scaffolding protein NHERF1 (Na^+/H^+ exchanger regulatory factor 1) is a regulator of sodium-hydrogen antiporter 3. It is encoded by the gene SLC9A3R1. It is also known as EBP50 (ERM Binding Protein 50) or SHAP3R1 (sodium-hydrogen antiporter 3 regulator 1). NHERF1 is composed of two tandem PSD-95/Drosophila discs large/ZO-1 (PDZ) protein interaction domains (PDZ1-PDZ2) in the N-terminus, and a C-terminal domain that binds the ezrin-radixinmoesi--merlin (ERM) family of cytoskeletal proteins. It is believed to interact *via* long-range allostery, involving significant protein dynamics [126]. NHERF1 has been reported to associated with several GPCRs such as β2-adrenergic receptor (β2AR) [127, 128], the κ-opioid receptor (κ-OR) [129], as well as growth factor tyrosine kinase receptors such as the platelet-derived growth factor receptor (PDGFR) [130] and the epidermal growth factor receptor (EGFR) [131]. In our previous work, we identified that NHERF1 also interact with HIV-1 co-receptor CCR5

[122]. Intriguingly, an increasing evidence revealed that PDZ and ERM domain-containing proteins are involved in the regulation of retroviral replication [132 - 134].

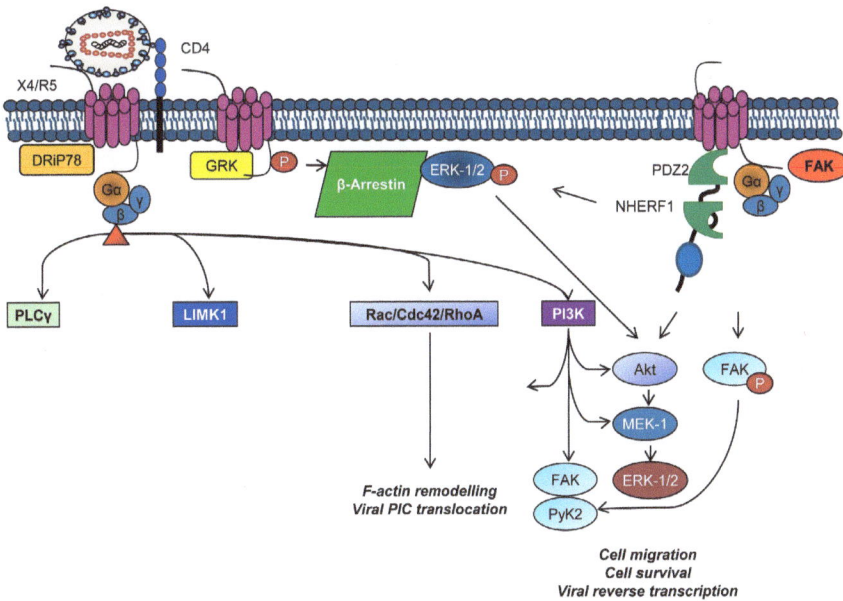

Fig. (12). HIV-1 co-receptors internalization and interacting proteins.

NHERF1 was identified to regulate the processes of HIV-1 entry and replication. A recent study suggests that CCR5 internalization can be promoted by NHERF1 upon stimulation with gp120 or RANTES, NHERF1 knockdown can increase CCR5 surface expression while NHERF1 overexpression can decrease CCR5 surface expression [122]. We used human osteosarcoma cells co-expressing CD4 and CCR5 (HOS-CD4-CCR5) cells to analyze effects of NHERF1 in different aspects of HIV-1 infection. In M-tropic HIV-1 infection, WT-NHERF1 overexpression can increase HIV-1 infection and replication while ERM, PDZ2 and PDZ1-PDZ2 fragments of NHERF1 overexpression can inhibit HIV-1 replication. In CCR5 interaction, NHERF1 can be recruited to CCR5 following stimulation by gp120 but interact weakly with CCR5. In MAPK/ERK and FAK signaling pathway regulation, both wild type NHERF1 and ERM domain of NHERF1 are able to promote ERK-1/2 and FAK phosphorylation, while PDZ1, PDZ2 of NHERF1 can increase ERK-1/2 phosphorylation and PDZ2-ERM can increase FAK phosphorylation. This activation is helpful for HIV-1 infection because MAPK/ERK signaling pathway can stimulate HIV-1 reverse transcription and FAK signaling pathway influences cell adhesion and migration [40, 135]. In filamentous actin and RhoA, gp120-induced CCR5 stimulation impels NHERF1 to strengthen the rearrangement of actin filament in host cells as well as potentiate RhoA (Ras homolog gene family member A) activations which are involved in HIV-1 post-entry replication [136, 137].

DRiP78

DRiP78 (Dopamine Receptor-interacting Protein 78), also known as DnaJC14 (DnaJ (Hsp40) homolog, subfamily C, member 14) and Jiv, is a molecular chaperone, which can bind ER membrane. It regulates the transport to plasma membrane of various 7TM-Rs including D1 dopamine receptor, M2 muscarinic acetylcholine receptor, and AT1 angiotensin II receptor [138, 139]. We also identified that DRiP78 interacts with homodimers of CXCR4 and CCR5 and facilitate the formation of homodimers complex, but cannot act on the heterodimer of CCR5-CXCR4 [75]. CXCR4 and CCR5 share part of a DRiP78-recognition sequence (F/L(x)3, 4FxxxF). GPCRs like D1-dopamine, M2-Muscarinic, A1-Adenosine, D2-dopamine and β2-adrenergic receptors which can interact with DRiP78 all share this sequence in the C-terminal tail [138 - 140]. Obviously, the DRiP78-recognition sequence plays a significant role in co-receptor-interaction. DRiP78 overexpression causes receptor localization from the plasma membrane to ER (endoplasmic reticulum) compartments change which results in the reduction of CCR5 localization to the plasma membrane [123, 137]. DRiP78 is considered as an HIV-1 co-receptor-interacting molecule taking account of the DRiP78's influence in these aspects, especially in CCR5 and CXCR4. Last year, HIV-1 model GHOST(3) cell line with DRiP78 or NHERF1 knockdown was established. We designed short hairpin RNA (shRNA) to construct DRiP78 or NHERF1 shRNA-expressing lentiviral vector in order to silence DRiP78 or NHERF1 gene expression. In the lentiviral vectors expressing DRiP78 or NHERF1 shRNA in the GHOST(3)-CXCR4 and GHOST(3)-CCR5 cell lines, the western blot analysis showed that DRiP78 and NHERF1 gene expression decreased 89.75% and 79.69% in GHOST(3)-CXCR4 cell line, decreased 78.29% and 74.55% in GHOST(3)-CCR5 cell line respectively. These findings prove that utilizing lentiviral vectors to carry shRNA is an optimal choice to silence a target gene. DRiP78 shRNA GHOST(3) cell line was used to identify the function of DRiP78 in HIV-1 infection and replication and the result show DRiP78 gene silencing can abrogate the replication of HIV-1 [137, 141]. It has also been shown that aberrant expression of DRiP78 results in the replication inhibition of yellow fever virus (YFV), which is mdediated by the interaction with a viral transmembrane domain (TMD) and a membrane-binding domain (MBD) [142, 143].

In summary, considering the particular effects of DRiP78 and NHERF1 in HIV-1infection process, small molecules or domain-derived peptides could aid to develop novel HIV-1 antagonists in the future.

CONCLUSION

Entry inhibitors are a new class of antiretroviral drugs. This class of drugs interferes with the binding, fusion and entry of an HIV virion to a human cell. By blocking this step in HIV's replication cycle, such agents slow the progression from HIV infection to AIDS. This chapter provides a comprehensive, up to date discussion of the current state of knowledge and the ongoing fundamental and applied research related to chemokine receptor-based anti-HIV-1 drugs. It is clear that much has been learned in preclinical development and clinical successes of co-receptors antagonists, especially with regard to CCR5. It is imperative to improve our limited understanding of the fundamental, complex processes that determine the co-receptor involved HIV-1 infection, and to apply these understandings to the development of safer and more effective next generation candidates for HIV/AIDS treatment and prophylactic strategies.

CONSENT FOR PUBLICATION

Not applicable.

CONFLICT OF INTEREST

The author (editor) declares no conflict of interest, financial or otherwise.

ACKNOWLEDGEMENTS

This work was supported by the National Natural Science Foundation of China (grants No. 31200130 and 81371812) and the Fund for Creative Talent of Science and Technology in University of Henan Province, China (grant No. 17HASTIT049). The author wish to thank Miss Jing Wen for preparing the manuscript, and Dr. Xin Yan for critical review of the manuscript.

REFERENCES

[1]   Hammer SM, Saag MS, Schechter M, Montaner JS, Schooley RT, Jacobsen DM, *et al.* Treatment for adult HIV infection: 2006 recommendations of the International AIDS Society-USA panel. JAMA 2006; 296: 827-43.

[2]   Kuhmann SE, Hartley O. Targeting chemokine receptors in HIV: a status report. Annu Rev Pharmacol Toxicol 2008; 48: 425-61.

[3]   Eckert DM, Kim PS. Design of potent inhibitors of HIV-1 entry from the gp41 N-peptide region. Proc Natl Acad Sci USA 2001; 98: 11187-92.

[4]   Roche M, Salimi H, Duncan R, Wilkinson BL, Chikere K, Moore MS, *et al.* A common mechanism of

clinical HIV-1 resistance to the CCR5 antagonist maraviroc despite divergent resistance levels and lack of common gp120 resistance mutations. Retrovirology 2013; 10: 43.

[5]   Weiss RA. Thirty years on: HIV receptor gymnastics and the prevention of infection. BMC Biol 2013; 11: 57.

[6]   Connor RI, Sheridan KE, Ceradini D, Choe S, Landau NR. Change in coreceptor use correlates with disease progression in HIV-1--infected individuals. J Exp Med 1997; 185: 621-8.

[7]   Hutter G, Bodor J, Ledger S, *et al.* CCR5 Targeted Cell Therapy for HIV and Prevention of Viral Escape. Viruses 2015; 7: 4186-203.

[8]   Wilen CB, Tilton JC, Doms RW. Molecular mechanisms of HIV entry. Adv Exp Med Biol 2012; 726: 223-42.

[9]   Watson C, Jenkinson S, Kazmierski W, Kenakin T. The CCR5 receptor-based mechanism of action of 873140, a potent allosteric noncompetitive HIV entry inhibitor. Mol Pharmacol 2005; 67: 1268-82.

[10]   Gu WG, Chen XQ. Targeting CCR5 for anti-HIV research. Eur J Clin Microbiol Infect Dis 2014; 33: 1881-7.

[11]   Van Der Ryst E. Maraviroc - A CCR5 Antagonist for the Treatment of HIV-1 Infection. Front Immunol 2015; 6: 277.

[12]   Dorr P, Westby M, Dobbs S, *et al.* Maraviroc (UK-427,857), a potent, orally bioavailable, and selective small-molecule inhibitor of chemokine receptor CCR5 with broad-spectrum anti-human immunodeficiency virus type 1 activity. Antimicrob Agents Chemother 2005; 49: 4721-32.

[13]   Jacobson JM, Lalezari JP, Thompson MA, *et al.* Phase 2a study of the CCR5 monoclonal antibody PRO 140 administered intravenously to HIV-infected adults. Antimicrob Agents Chemother 2010; 54: 4137-42.

[14]   Jacobson JM, Thompson MA, Lalezari JP, *et al.* Anti-HIV-1 activity of weekly or biweekly treatment with subcutaneous PRO 140, a CCR5 monoclonal antibody. J Infect Dis 2010; 201: 1481-7.

[15]   Giroud C, Marin M, Hammonds J, Spearman P, Melikyan GB. P2X1 Receptor Antagonists Inhibit HIV-1 Fusion by Blocking Virus-Coreceptor Interactions. J Virol 2015; 89: 9368-82.

[16]   Feng Y, Broder CC, Kennedy PE, Berger EA. HIV-1 entry cofactor: functional cDNA cloning of a seven-transmembrane, G protein-coupled receptor. Science 1996; 272: 872-7.

[17]   Berger EA, Murphy PM, Farber JM. Chemokine receptors as HIV-1 coreceptors: roles in viral entry, tropism, and disease. Annu Rev Immunol 1999; 17: 657-700.

[18]   Tsao LC, Guo H, Jeffrey J, Hoxie JA, Su L. CCR5 interaction with HIV-1 Env contributes to Env-induced depletion of CD4 T cells *in vitro* and *in vivo*. Retrovirology 2016; 13: 22.

[19]   Wu Y, Yoder A. Chemokine coreceptor signaling in HIV-1 infection and pathogenesis. PLoS Pathog 2009; 5: e1000520.

[20]   Murphy PM. Chemokine receptors: structure, function and role in microbial pathogenesis. Cytokine Growth Factor Rev 1996; 7: 47-64.

[21]   Davis CB, Dikic I, Unutmaz D, *et al.* Signal transduction due to HIV-1 envelope interactions with chemokine receptors CXCR4 or CCR5. J Exp Med 1997; 186: 1793-8.

[22]   Abbas W, Herbein G. Plasma membrane signaling in HIV-1 infection. Biochim Biophys Acta 2014; 1838: 1132-42.

[23]   Kinter A, Catanzaro A, Monaco J, *et al.* CC-chemokines enhance the replication of T-tropic strains of HIV-1 in CD4(+) T cells: role of signal transduction. Proc Natl Acad Sci USA 1998; 95: 11880-5.

[24]   Chackerian B, Long EM, Luciw PA, Overbaugh J. Human immunodeficiency virus type 1 coreceptors participate in postentry stages in the virus replication cycle and function in simian immunodeficiency virus infection. J Virol 1997; 71: 3932-9.

[25] Kelly MD, Naif HM, Adams SL, Cunningham AL, Lloyd AR. Dichotomous effects of beta-chemokines on HIV replication in monocytes and monocyte-derived macrophages. J Immunol 1998; 160: 3091-5.

[26] Cocchi F, DeVico AL, Garzino-Demo A, Cara A, Gallo RC, Lusso P. The V3 domain of the HIV-1 gp120 envelope glycoprotein is critical for chemokine-mediated blockade of infection. Nat Med 1996; 2: 1244-7.

[27] Yoder A, Yu D, Dong L, *et al.* HIV envelope-CXCR4 signaling activates cofilin to overcome cortical actin restriction in resting CD4 T cells. Cell 2008; 134: 782-92.

[28] Desmetz C, Lin YL, Mettling C, *et al.* The strength of the chemotactic response to a CCR5 binding chemokine is determined by the level of cell surface CCR5 density. Immunology 2006; 119: 551-61.

[29] Del Corno M, Liu QH, Schols D, *et al.* HIV-1 gp120 and chemokine activation of Pyk2 and mitogen-activated protein kinases in primary macrophages mediated by calcium-dependent, pertussis toxin-insensitive chemokine receptor signaling. Blood 2001; 98: 2909-16.

[30] Reckless J, Grainger DJ. Identification of oligopeptide sequences which inhibit migration induced by a wide range of chemokines. Biochem J 1999; 340(Pt 3): 803-11.

[31] Grainger DJ, Reckless J. Broad-spectrum chemokine inhibitors (BSCIs) and their anti-inflammatory effects *in vivo*. Biochem Pharmacol 2003; 65: 1027-34.

[32] Grainger DJ, Lever AM. Blockade of chemokine-induced signalling inhibits CCR5-dependent HIV infection *in vitro* without blocking gp120/CCR5 interaction. Retrovirology 2005; 2: 23.

[33] Paruch S, Heinis M, Lemay J, *et al.* CCR5 signaling through phospholipase D involves p44/42 MAP-kinases and promotes HIV-1 LTR-directed gene expression. FASEB J 2007; 21: 4038-46.

[34] Francois F, Klotman ME. Phosphatidylinositol 3-kinase regulates human immunodeficiency virus type 1 replication following viral entry in primary CD4+ T lymphocytes and macrophages. J Virol 2003; 77: 2539-49.

[35] Lin YL, Mettling C, Portales P, Reynes J, Clot J, Corbeau P. Cell surface CCR5 density determines the postentry efficiency of R5 HIV-1 infection. Proc Natl Acad Sci USA 2002; 99: 15590-5.

[36] Lin YL, Mettling C, Portales P, Reant B, Clot J, Corbeau P. G-protein signaling triggered by R5 human immunodeficiency virus type 1 increases virus replication efficiency in primary T lymphocytes. J Virol 2005; 79: 7938-41.

[37] Lin YL, Mettling C, Portales P, *et al.* The efficiency of R5 HIV-1 infection is determined by CD4 T-cell surface CCR5 density through G alpha i-protein signalling. AIDS 2006; 20: 1369-77.

[38] Kinet S, Bernard F, Mongellaz C, Perreau M, Goldman FD, Taylor N. gp120-mediated induction of the MAPK cascade is dependent on the activation state of CD4(+) lymphocytes. Blood 2002; 100: 2546-53.

[39] Amella CA, Sherry B, Shepp DH, Schmidtmayerova H. Macrophage inflammatory protein 1alpha inhibits postentry steps of human immunodeficiency virus type 1 infection *via* suppression of intracellular cyclic AMP. J Virol 2005; 79: 5625-31.

[40] Mettling C, Desmetz C, Fiser AL, Reant B, Corbeau P, Lin YL. Galphai protein-dependant extracellular signal-regulated kinase-1/2 activation is required for HIV-1 reverse transcription. AIDS 2008; 22: 1569-76.

[41] Popik W, Hesselgesser JE, Pitha PM. Binding of human immunodeficiency virus type 1 to CD4 and CXCR4 receptors differentially regulates expression of inflammatory genes and activates the MEK/ERK signaling pathway. J Virol 1998; 72: 6406-13.

[42] Popik W, Pitha PM. Exploitation of cellular signaling by HIV-1: unwelcome guests with master keys that signal their entry. Virology 2000; 276: 1-6.

[43] Misse D, Cerutti M, Noraz N, *et al.* A CD4-independent interaction of human immunodeficiency

virus-1 gp120 with CXCR4 induces their cointernalization, cell signaling, and T-cell chemotaxis. Blood 1999; 93: 2454-62.

[44] Montes M, Tagieva NE, Heveker N, Nahmias C, Baleux F, Trautmann A. SDF-1-induced activation of ERK enhances HIV-1 expression. Eur Cytokine Netw 2000; 11: 470-7.

[45] Guntermann C, Murphy BJ, Zheng R, Qureshi A, Eagles PA, Nye KE. Human immunodeficiency virus-1 infection requires pertussis toxin sensitive G-protein-coupled signalling and mediates cAMP downregulation. Biochem Biophys Res Commun 1999; 256: 429-35.

[46] Misse D, Gajardo J, Oblet C, et al. Soluble HIV-1 gp120 enhances HIV-1 replication in non-dividing CD4+ T cells, mediated *via* cell signaling and Tat cofactor overexpression. AIDS 2005; 19: 897-905.

[47] Tan Q, Zhu Y, Li J, et al. Structure of the CCR5 chemokine receptor-HIV entry inhibitor maraviroc complex. Science 2013; 341: 1387-90.

[48] Doranz BJ, Lu ZH, Rucker J, et al. Two distinct CCR5 domains can mediate coreceptor usage by human immunodeficiency virus type 1. J Virol 1997; 71: 6305-14.

[49] Huang CC, Lam SN, Acharya P, et al. Structures of the CCR5 N terminus and of a tyrosine-sulfated antibody with HIV-1 gp120 and CD4. Science 2007; 317: 1930-4.

[50] Duma L, Haussinger D, Rogowski M, Lusso P, Grzesiek S. Recognition of RANTES by extracellular parts of the CCR5 receptor. J Mol Biol 2007; 365: 1063-75.

[51] Combadiere C, Ahuja SK, Tiffany HL, Murphy PM. Cloning and functional expression of CC CKR5, a human monocyte CC chemokine receptor selective for MIP-1(alpha), MIP-1(beta), and RANTES. J Leukoc Biol 1996; 60: 147-52.

[52] Samson M, Labbe O, Mollereau C, Vassart G, Parmentier M. Molecular cloning and functional expression of a new human CC-chemokine receptor gene. Biochemistry 1996; 35: 3362-7.

[53] Blanpain C, Migeotte I, Lee B, et al. CCR5 binds multiple CC-chemokines: MCP-3 acts as a natural antagonist. Blood 1999; 94: 1899-905.

[54] Cocchi F, DeVico AL, Garzino-Demo A, Arya SK, Gallo RC, Lusso P. Identification of RANTES, MIP-1 alpha, and MIP-1 beta as the major HIV-suppressive factors produced by CD8+ T cells. Science 1995; 270: 1811-5.

[55] Ansari AW, Heiken H, Moenkemeyer M, Schmidt RE. Dichotomous effects of C-C chemokines in HIV-1 pathogenesis. Immunol Lett 2007; 110: 1-5.

[56] Miyakawa T, Obaru K, Maeda K, Harada S, Mitsuya H. Identification of amino acid residues critical for LD78beta, a variant of human macrophage inflammatory protein-1alpha, binding to CCR5 and inhibition of R5 human immunodeficiency virus type 1 replication. J Biol Chem 2002; 277: 4649-55.

[57] Seibert C, Ying W, Gavrilov S, et al. Interaction of small molecule inhibitors of HIV-1 entry with CCR5. Virology 2006; 349: 41-54.

[58] Cormier EG, Persuh M, Thompson DA, et al. Specific interaction of CCR5 amino-terminal domain peptides containing sulfotyrosines with HIV-1 envelope glycoprotein gp120. Proc Natl Acad Sci USA 2000; 97: 5762-7.

[59] Farzan M, Mirzabekov T, Kolchinsky P, et al. Tyrosine sulfation of the amino terminus of CCR5 facilitates HIV-1 entry. Cell 1999; 96: 667-76.

[60] Castonguay LA, Weng Y, Adolfsen W, et al. Binding of 2-aryl-4-(piperidin-1-yl)butanamines and 1,3,4-trisubstituted pyrrolidines to human CCR5: a molecular modeling-guided mutagenesis study of the binding pocket. Biochemistry 2003; 42: 1544-50.

[61] Dragic T, Trkola A, Thompson DA, et al. A binding pocket for a small molecule inhibitor of HIV-1 entry within the transmembrane helices of CCR5. Proc Natl Acad Sci USA 2000; 97: 5639-44.

[62] Nishikawa M, Takashima K, Nishi T, et al. Analysis of binding sites for the new small-molecule CCR5 antagonist TAK-220 on human CCR5. Antimicrob Agents Chemother 2005; 49: 4708-15.

[63]   Tsamis F, Gavrilov S, Kajumo F, *et al.* Analysis of the mechanism by which the small-molecule CCR5 antagonists SCH-351125 and SCH-350581 inhibit human immunodeficiency virus type 1 entry. J Virol 2003; 77: 5201-8.

[64]   Maeda K, Das D, Ogata-Aoki H, *et al.* Structural and molecular interactions of CCR5 inhibitors with CCR5. J Biol Chem 2006; 281: 12688-98.

[65]   Olson WC, Jacobson JM. CCR5 monoclonal antibodies for HIV-1 therapy. Curr Opin HIV AIDS 2009; 4: 104-11.

[66]   Samson M, Libert F, Doranz BJ, *et al.* Resistance to HIV-1 infection in caucasian individuals bearing mutant alleles of the CCR-5 chemokine receptor gene. Nature 1996; 382: 722-5.

[67]   Pasi KJ, Sabin CA, Jenkins PV, Devereux HL, Ononye C, Lee CA. The effects of the 32-bp CCR-5 deletion on HIV transmission and HIV disease progression in individuals with haemophilia. Br J Haematol 2000; 111: 136-42.

[68]   Wilkin TJ, Gulick RM. CCR5 antagonism in HIV infection: current concepts and future opportunities. Annu Rev Med 2012; 63: 81-93.

[69]   Mueller A, Mahmoud NG, Goedecke MC, McKeating JA, Strange PG. Pharmacological characterization of the chemokine receptor, CCR5. Br J Pharmacol 2002; 135: 1033-43.

[70]   Rosario MC, Jacqmin P, Dorr P, *et al.* Population pharmacokinetic/pharmacodynamic analysis of CCR5 receptor occupancy by maraviroc in healthy subjects and HIV-positive patients. Br J Clin Pharmacol 2008; 65 (Suppl. 1): 86-94.

[71]   Fatkenheuer G, Pozniak AL, Johnson MA, *et al.* Efficacy of short-term monotherapy with maraviroc, a new CCR5 antagonist, in patients infected with HIV-1. Nat Med 2005; 11: 1170-2.

[72]   Westby M, Lewis M, Whitcomb J, *et al.* Emergence of CXCR4-using human immunodeficiency virus type 1 (HIV-1) variants in a minority of HIV-1-infected patients following treatment with the CCR5 antagonist maraviroc is from a pretreatment CXCR4-using virus reservoir. J Virol 2006; 80: 4909-20.

[73]   Gulick RM, Fatkenheuer G, Burnside R, *et al.* Five-year safety evaluation of maraviroc in HIV-infected treatment-experienced patients. J Acquir Immune Defic Syndr 2014; 65: 78-81.

[74]   Gulick RM, Lalezari J, Goodrich J, *et al.* Maraviroc for previously treated patients with R5 HIV-1 infection. N Engl J Med 2008; 359: 1429-41.

[75]   Hardy WD, Gulick RM, Mayer H, *et al.* Two-year safety and virologic efficacy of maraviroc in treatment-experienced patients with CCR5-tropic HIV-1 infection: 96-week combined analysis of MOTIVATE 1 and 2. J Acquir Immune Defic Syndr 2010; 55: 558-64.

[76]   Zhang J, Gao X, Martin J, *et al.* Evolution of coreceptor utilization to escape CCR5 antagonist therapy. Virology 2016; 494: 198-214.

[77]   Kim MB, Giesler KE, Tahirovic YA, Truax VM, Liotta DC, Wilson LJ. CCR5 receptor antagonists in preclinical to phase II clinical development for treatment of HIV. Expert Opin Investig Drugs 2016; 25: 1377-92.

[78]   Baba M, Takashima K, Miyake H, *et al.* TAK-652 inhibits CCR5-mediated human immunodeficiency virus type 1 infection *in vitro* and has favorable pharmacokinetics in humans. Antimicrob Agents Chemother 2005; 49: 4584-91.

[79]   Briz V, Poveda E, Soriano V. HIV entry inhibitors: mechanisms of action and resistance pathways. J Antimicrob Chemother 2006; 57: 619-27.

[80]   Marier JF, Trinh M, Pheng LH, Palleja SM, Martin DE. Pharmacokinetics and pharmacodynamics of TBR-652, a novel CCR5 antagonist, in HIV-1-infected, antiretroviral treatment-experienced, CCR5 antagonist-naive patients. Antimicrob Agents Chemother 2011; 55: 2768-74.

[81]   Klibanov OM, Williams SH, Iler CA. Cenicriviroc, an orally active CCR5 antagonist for the potential treatment of HIV infection. Curr Opin Investig Drugs 2010; 11: 940-50.

[82]   Ratziu V. Novel Pharmacotherapy Options for NASH. Dig Dis Sci 2016; 61: 1398-405.

[83]   Kagan RM, Johnson EP, Siaw MF, *et al.* Comparison of genotypic and phenotypic HIV type 1 tropism assay: results from the screening samples of Cenicriviroc Study 202, a randomized phase II trial in treatment-naive subjects. AIDS Res Hum Retroviruses 2014; 30: 151-9.

[84]   Baba M, Miyake H, Wang X, Okamoto M, Takashima K. Isolation and characterization of human immunodeficiency virus type 1 resistant to the small-molecule CCR5 antagonist TAK-652. Antimicrob Agents Chemother 2007; 51: 707-15.

[85]   Thompson M, Saag M, DeJesus E, *et al.* A 48-week randomized phase 2b study evaluating cenicriviroc *versus* efavirenz in treatment-naive HIV-infected adults with C-C chemokine receptor type 5-tropic virus. AIDS 2016; 30: 869-78.

[86]   Brown KC, Paul S, Kashuba AD. Drug interactions with new and investigational antiretrovirals. Clin Pharmacokinet 2009; 48: 211-41.

[87]   Shin N, Solomon K, Zhou N, *et al.* Identification and characterization of INCB9471, an allosteric noncompetitive small-molecule antagonist of C-C chemokine receptor 5 with potent inhibitory activity against monocyte migration and HIV-1 infection. J Pharmacol Exp Ther 2011; 338: 228-39.

[88]   Cohen C, DeJesus E, Mills A, *et al.* Potent antiretroviral activity of the once-daily CCR5 antagonist INCB009471 over 14 days of monotherapy 4th IAS Conference on AIDS Pathogenesis, Treatment and Prevention. 22-5.

[89]   Erickson-Viitanen S, Ambremski K, Solomon K. Co-receptor tropism, ENV genotype, and *in vitro* susceptibility to CCR5 antagonists during a 14-day monotherapy study with INCB9471 15th Conference on Retroviruses and Opportunistic Infections. 3-6.

[90]   Polianova MT, Ruscetti FW, Pert CB, Ruff MR. Chemokine receptor-5 (CCR5) is a receptor for the HIV entry inhibitor peptide T (DAPTA). Antiviral Res 2005; 67: 83-92.

[91]   Pollicita M, Ruff MR, Pert CB, *et al.* Profound anti-HIV-1 activity of DAPTA in monocytes/macrophages and inhibition of CCR5-mediated apoptosis in neuronal cells. Antivir Chem Chemother 2007; 18: 285-95.

[92]   Goodkin K, Vitiello B, Lyman WD, *et al.* Cerebrospinal and peripheral human immunodeficiency virus type 1 load in a multisite, randomized, double-blind, placebo-controlled trial of D-Ala1-peptide T-amide for HIV-1-associated cognitive-motor impairment. J Neurovirol 2006; 12: 178-89.

[93]   Ruff MR, Smith C, Kingan T, *et al.* Pharmacokinetics of peptide T in patients with acquired immunodeficiency syndrome (AIDS). Prog Neuropsychopharmacol Biol Psychiatry 1991; 15: 791-801.

[94]   Polianova MT, Ruscetti FW, Pert CB, *et al.* Antiviral and immunological benefits in HIV patients receiving intranasal peptide T (DAPTA). Peptides 2003; 24: 1093-8.

[95]   Emmelkamp JM, Rockstroh JK. CCR5 antagonists: comparison of efficacy, side effects, pharmacokinetics and interactions--review of the literature. Eur J Med Res 2007; 12: 409-17.

[96]   Strizki JM, Tremblay C, Xu S, *et al.* Discovery and characterization of vicriviroc (SCH 417690), a CCR5 antagonist with potent activity against human immunodeficiency virus type 1. Antimicrob Agents Chemother 2005; 49: 4911-9.

[97]   Kasserra C, O'Mara E. Pharmacokinetic interaction of vicriviroc with other antiretroviral agents: results from a series of fixed-sequence and parallel-group clinical trials. Clin Pharmacokinet 2011; 50: 267-80.

[98]   McNicholas P, Vilchez RA, Greaves W, *et al.* Detection of HIV-1 CXCR4 tropism and resistance in treatment experienced subjects receiving CCR5 antagonist-Vicriviroc. J Clin Virol 2012; 55: 134-9.

[99]   Asin-Milan O, Chamberland A, Wei Y, Haidara A, Sylla M, Tremblay CL. Mutations in variable domains of the HIV-1 envelope gene can have a significant impact on maraviroc and vicriviroc

resistance. AIDS Res Ther 2013; 10: 15.

[100]   Anastassopoulou CG, Ketas TJ, Sanders RW, Klasse PJ, Moore JP. Effects of sequence changes in the HIV-1 gp41 fusion peptide on CCR5 inhibitor resistance. Virology 2012; 428: 86-97.

[101]   Olson WC, Rabut GE, Nagashima KA, *et al.* Differential inhibition of human immunodeficiency virus type 1 fusion, gp120 binding, and CC-chemokine activity by monoclonal antibodies to CCR5. J Virol 1999; 73: 4145-55.

[102]   Murga JD, Franti M, Pevear DC, Maddon PJ, Olson WC. Potent antiviral synergy between monoclonal antibody and small-molecule CCR5 inhibitors of human immunodeficiency virus type 1. Antimicrob Agents Chemother 2006; 50: 3289-96.

[103]   Jacobson JM, Saag MS, Thompson MA, *et al.* Antiviral activity of single-dose PRO 140, a CCR5 monoclonal antibody, in HIV-infected adults. J Infect Dis 2008; 198: 1345-52.

[104]   Federsppiel B, Melhado IG, Duncan AM, *et al.* Molecular cloning of the cDNA and chromosomal localization of the gene for a putative seven-transmembrane segment (7-TMS) receptor isolated from human spleen. Genomics 1993; 16: 707-12.

[105]   Herzog H, Hort YJ, Shine J, Selbie LA. Molecular cloning, characterization, and localization of the human homolog to the reported bovine NPY Y3 receptor: lack of NPY binding and activation. DNA Cell Biol 1993; 12: 465-71.

[106]   Jazin EE, Yoo H, Blomqvist AG, *et al.* A proposed bovine neuropeptide Y (NPY) receptor cDNA clone, or its human homologue, confers neither NPY binding sites nor NPY responsiveness on transfected cells. Regul Pept 1993; 47: 247-58.

[107]   Loetscher M, Geiser T, O'Reilly T, Zwahlen R, Baggiolini M, Moser B. Cloning of a human seven-transmembrane domain receptor, LESTR, that is highly expressed in leukocytes. J Biol Chem 1994; 269: 232-7.

[108]   Nomura H, Nielsen BW, Matsushima K. Molecular cloning of cDNAs encoding a LD78 receptor and putative leukocyte chemotactic peptide receptors. Int Immunol 1993; 5: 1239-49.

[109]   Bleul CC, Farzan M, Choe H, *et al.* The lymphocyte chemoattractant SDF-1 is a ligand for LESTR/fusin and blocks HIV-1 entry. Nature 1996; 382: 829-33.

[110]   Oberlin E, Amara A, Bachelerie F, *et al.* The CXC chemokine SDF-1 is the ligand for LESTR/fusin and prevents infection by T-cell-line-adapted HIV-1. Nature 1996; 382: 833-5.

[111]   Yu L, Cecil J, Peng SB, *et al.* Identification and expression of novel isoforms of human stromal cell-derived factor 1. Gene 2006; 374: 174-9.

[112]   Altenburg JD, Broxmeyer HE, Jin Q, Cooper S, Basu S, Alkhatib G. A naturally occurring splice variant of CXCL12/stromal cell-derived factor 1 is a potent human immunodeficiency virus type 1 inhibitor with weak chemotaxis and cell survival activities. J Virol 2007; 81: 8140-8.

[113]   Broxmeyer HE, Orschell CM, Clapp DW, *et al.* Rapid mobilization of murine and human hematopoietic stem and progenitor cells with AMD3100, a CXCR4 antagonist. J Exp Med 2005; 201: 1307-18.

[114]   Jujo K, Ii M, Sekiguchi H, *et al.* CXC-chemokine receptor 4 antagonist AMD3100 promotes cardiac functional recovery after ischemia/reperfusion injury *via* endothelial nitric oxide synthase-dependent mechanism. Circulation 2013; 127: 63-73.

[115]   Das D, Maeda K, Hayashi Y, *et al.* Insights into the mechanism of inhibition of CXCR4: identification of Piperidinylethanamine analogs as anti-HIV-1 inhibitors. Antimicrob Agents Chemother 2015; 59: 1895-904.

[116]   Cao YJ, Flexner CW, Dunaway S, *et al.* Effect of low-dose ritonavir on the pharmacokinetics of the CXCR4 antagonist AMD070 in healthy volunteers. Antimicrob Agents Chemother 2008; 52: 1630-4.

[117]   Stone ND, Dunaway SB, Flexner C, *et al.* Multiple-dose escalation study of the safety,

pharmacokinetics, and biologic activity of oral AMD070, a selective CXCR4 receptor inhibitor, in human subjects. Antimicrob Agents Chemother 2007; 51: 2351-8.

[118] Moyle G, DeJesus E, Boffito M, Wong RS, Gibney C, Badel K, *et al*. Proof of activity with AMD11070, an orally bioavailable inhibitor of CXCR4-tropic HIV type 1. Clin Infect Dis 2009; 48: 798-805.

[119] Marchese A. Endocytic trafficking of chemokine receptors. Curr Opin Cell Biol 2014; 27: 72-7.

[120] Moore CA, Milano SK, Benovic JL. Regulation of receptor trafficking by GRKs and arrestins. Annu Rev Physiol 2007; 69: 451-82.

[121] Shenoy SK, Lefkowitz RJ. beta-Arrestin-mediated receptor trafficking and signal transduction. Trends Pharmacol Sci 2011; 32: 521-33.

[122] Hammad MM, Kuang YQ, Yan R, Allen H, Dupre DJ. Na+/H+ exchanger regulatory factor-1 is involved in chemokine receptor homodimer CCR5 internalization and signal transduction but does not affect CXCR4 homodimer or CXCR4-CCR5 heterodimer. J Biol Chem 2010; 285: 34653-64.

[123] Kuang YQ, Charette N, Frazer J, *et al*. Dopamine receptor-interacting protein 78 acts as a molecular chaperone for CCR5 chemokine receptor signaling complex organization. PLoS One 2012; 7: e40522.

[124] Bonsch C, Munteanu M, Rossitto-Borlat I, Furstenberg A, Hartley O. Potent Anti-HIV Chemokine Analogs Direct Post-Endocytic Sorting of CCR5. PLoS One 2015; 10: e0125396.

[125] Spear M, Guo J, Wu Y. Novel anti-HIV therapeutics targeting chemokine receptors and actin regulatory pathways. Immunol Rev 2013; 256: 300-12.

[126] Farago B, Li J, Cornilescu G, Callaway DJ, Bu Z. Activation of nanoscale allosteric protein domain motion revealed by neutron spin echo spectroscopy. Biophys J 2010; 99: 3473-82.

[127] Hall RA, Premont RT, Chow CW, *et al*. The beta2-adrenergic receptor interacts with the Na+/H+-exchanger regulatory factor to control Na+/H+ exchange. Nature 1998; 392: 626-30.

[128] Hall RA, Ostedgaard LS, Premont RT, *et al*. A C-terminal motif found in the beta2-adrenergic receptor, P2Y1 receptor and cystic fibrosis transmembrane conductance regulator determines binding to the Na+/H+ exchanger regulatory factor family of PDZ proteins. Proc Natl Acad Sci USA 1998; 95: 8496-501.

[129] Li JG, Chen C, Liu-Chen LY. Ezrin-radixin-moesin-binding phosphoprotein-50/Na+/H+ exchanger regulatory factor (EBP50/NHERF) blocks U50,488H-induced down-regulation of the human kappa opioid receptor by enhancing its recycling rate. J Biol Chem 2002; 277: 27545-52.

[130] Maudsley S, Zamah AM, Rahman N, *et al*. Platelet-derived growth factor receptor association with Na(+)/H(+) exchanger regulatory factor potentiates receptor activity. Mol Cell Biol 2000; 20: 8352-63.

[131] Lazar CS, Cresson CM, Lauffenburger DA, Gill GN. The Na+/H+ exchanger regulatory factor stabilizes epidermal growth factor receptors at the cell surface. Mol Biol Cell 2004; 15: 5470-80.

[132] Haedicke J, de Los Santos K, Goff SP, Naghavi MH. The Ezrin-radixin-moesin family member ezrin regulates stable microtubule formation and retroviral infection. J Virol 2008; 82: 4665-70.

[133] Kubo Y, Yoshii H, Kamiyama H, *et al*. Ezrin, Radixin, and Moesin (ERM) proteins function as pleiotropic regulators of human immunodeficiency virus type 1 infection. Virology 2008; 375: 130-40.

[134] Henning MS, Morham SG, Goff SP, Naghavi MH. PDZD8 is a novel Gag-interacting factor that promotes retroviral infection. J Virol 2010; 84: 8990-5.

[135] Frame MC, Patel H, Serrels B, Lietha D, Eck MJ. The FERM domain: organizing the structure and function of FAK. Nat Rev Mol Cell Biol 2010; 11: 802-14.

[136] Kuang YQ, Pang W, Zheng YT, Dupre DJ. NHERF1 regulates gp120-induced internalization and signaling by CCR5, and HIV-1 production. Eur J Immunol 2012; 42: 299-310.

[137] Zhang L, Huang XH, Zhou PP, *et al*. Establishment of HIV-1 model cell line GHOST(3) with stable

DRiP78 and NHERF1 knockdown. Dongwuxue Yanjiu 2015; 36: 161-6.

[138] Bermak JC, Li M, Bullock C, Zhou QY. Regulation of transport of the dopamine D1 receptor by a new membrane-associated ER protein. Nat Cell Biol 2001; 3: 492-8.

[139] Leclerc PC, Auger-Messier M, Lanctot PM, Escher E, Leduc R, Guillemette G. A polyaromatic caveolin-binding-like motif in the cytoplasmic tail of the type 1 receptor for angiotensin II plays an important role in receptor trafficking and signaling. Endocrinology 2002; 143: 4702-10.

[140] Dupre DJ, Robitaille M, Richer M, Ethier N, Mamarbachi AM, Hebert TE. Dopamine receptor-interacting protein 78 acts as a molecular chaperone for Ggamma subunits before assembly with Gbeta. J Biol Chem 2007; 282: 13703-15.

[141] Li C, Zhang YJ, Denis JD, Kuang YQ. Chemokine receptors and their interactors in HIV-1 replication: potential therapeutic targets. Receptors Clin Investig 2015.

[142] Yi Z, Sperzel L, Nurnberger C, *et al.* Identification and characterization of the host protein DNAJC14 as a broadly active flavivirus replication modulator. PLoS Pathog 2011; 7: e1001255.

[143] Yi Z, Yuan Z, Rice CM, MacDonald MR. Flavivirus replication complex assembly revealed by DNAJC14 functional mapping. J Virol 2012; 86: 11815-32.

CHAPTER 5

Sexually Transmitted Co-infections in Persons Living with HIV

Ana Paula Ferreira Costa, Marcos Gonzaga dos Santos and Ricardo Ney Oliveira Cobucci*

Avenida Salgado Filho, 1610, Natal-RN, 59056-000, Brazil

Abstract: Sexually transmitted co-infections increase HIV infectiousness through local inflammatory processes. The risk factors in acquiring genital co-infections associated with HIV infection still present many questions. There is some evidence that there is an association between certain sexually transmitted infections and HIV, but for others, there is only a marginal correlation, as will be discussed in this chapter. The most prevalent co-infections found in HIV carriers and their epidemiology, clinical features and evidence-based treatments will also be analyzed.

Keywords: Acquired Immune Deficiency Syndrome Virus, *Chlamydia trachomatis*, Human Immunodeficiency Virus, HSV, HPV, *Neisseria gonorrhoeae*, Sexually Transmitted Infections, Syphilis, *Trichomonas vaginalis*.

1. HIV – BACKGROUND

The Human Immunodeficiency virus (HIV), which causes the Acquired Immunodeficiency Syndrome (AIDS), appeared in mid-1981 in the United States, causing serious damage to the immune system of infected individuals. As the virus destroys immune CD4+ T-cells, the individual becomes progressively immunodeficient [1, 2]. Despite all the advances in the field, HIV continues to be a major global public health issue and the World Health Organization estimates that one million people died from HIV in 2016.

With the use of antiretroviral therapy (ART), HIV infection came to be considered a chronic condition that could be controlled, which resulted in the improvement of morbidity indicators with a reduction in opportunistic diseases. There is also increasing evidence that early ART can markedly reduce the risk of sexual transmission to HIV-negative sexual partners among heterosexual couples. This suggests that the "treatment as prevention" approach could be used as part of a

---

* Corresponding author Ricardo Ney Oliveira Cobucci: Avenida Salgado Filho, 1610, Natal - RN, Zip code 59056-000, Brazil, Tel: +558432151234, E-mail address: rncobucci@hotmail.com

Atta-ur-Rahman (Ed.)

strategy to prevent the epidemic [3 - 6]. However, as ART has enhanced the quality of life and sexual health, the transmission of Sexually Transmitted Infections (STIs) has also increased. There is also the fact that individuals living with HIV, and those at risk can prevent transmission without the use of a barrier method of protection and this motivates decreased condom use [7].

The subsequent longevity also contributed to the appearance of other health problems, either due to the prolonged effect of therapy and the concomitance of drug toxicity or the appearance of comorbidities and/or treatment-resistant viral variants [8]. Furthermore, the diversity of partners, favors a predisposition to STIs. Low immunity in HIV-positive individuals facilitates the entry of new opportunistic microorganisms, spreading the infection, especially during unprotected sex, favoring the emergence of viral infections such as HPV, HSV and/or bacterial infections.

Clinical and epidemiological studies showed a positive correlation between STIs and increased genital tract shedding and/or susceptibility to HIV infection [9, 10]. HIV infected women also bearing STI, have an increased viral load in genital secretions, potentially increasing the chance of transmission [11, 12].Therefore, the purpose of this chapter is to address the most prevalent genital infections among HIV carriers.

2. VIRAL GENITAL INFECTIONS

2.1. Human Papillomavirus (HPV)

Human papillomaviruses (HPV) are DNA viruses that infect basal epithelial (skin or mucosal) cells [13]. HPV is recognized as one of the most common sexually transmitted infections. HPV type 6 and 11 have been associated with warts [14], while others, like 16 and 18, have been well established as the main risk factors of invasive cervical cancers and their associated pre-cancerous lesions, such as those found in the cervix, vulva, vagina, penis, anus, rectum and oropharynx [15].

HPV detection in the absence of apparent disease is found in 11–12% of all women. Detection is higher in young women (50–80%) and declines at an older age. Such unapparent infections are typically characterized by multiple HPV types, including HPV 16 (3.2%), 18 (1.4%), 31 (0.8%), and 58 (0.7%). HPV detection increases with disease severity, with a percentage of positivity in cervical intraepithelial neoplasia 1 (CIN1) at 50 –70%, CIN2 has (85%) positivity for HPV and in CIN3 and invasive cervical cancer the positivity rises to between (90% - 100%) [11].

HPV infection is commonly found among HIV-positive individuals. The prevalence of HPV infections is greatest among individuals infected with HIV, ranging from 40% to 93%. The prevalence of HPV infection was 67% among women HIV carriers, with a lower propensity to eliminate this virus, increasing the risk of developing lesions and cancer [10], however, it is higher in homosexual men [16]. Thus, the prevalence of anal HPV infection, tested with PCR, was 93% among HIV-positive subjects and 61% among HIV-negative subjects. The most common type was HPV 16, detected respectively in 38% and 19% of specimens [17].

Co-infection of genital HPV with HIV is biologically acceptable. Both viruses share the same mechanism of access to susceptible cells as the squamocolumnar junctions, a site predisposed to viral establishment. HPV causes the rupture of the integrity of the epithelium and mucosal immune system, facilitating the infection and spread of HIV, altering the functional activities of phagocytic epithelial cells, reducing the production of proteins involved in antimicrobial activities, and increasing the expression of inflammatory cytokines that facilitate HIV replication [18].

HIV and its connection with invasive cervical cancer dates from the earliest descriptions of AIDS. The low CD4+ T-cells count due to HIV-associated immunosuppression favors the increased risk of cervical cancer [19]. ART reduce opportunistic infections, but not the incidence of cervical carcinomas, probably due to the HPV latency phase [20]. The low number of CD4+ T-cells is associated with greater positivity of multiple HPV infections, which is consistent between users and non-users of ART [21]. However, favorable effects of prolonged use of ART on infection and cervical precancerous lesions are associated with the high number of CD4+ T-cells. The extended use of ART is necessary due to the long process of reestablishment of immunity that depends on different phases, such as the immediate redistribution of memory T cells followed by the expansion of naive T-cells, which are active against new pathogens [22].

The most important methods to diagnose HPV infection are:

- Pap smear: described by Papanicolaou and Traut and is a screening test. A positive test requires further confirmatory tests like coloscopy, cervical biopsy, and DNA tests like PCR.
- Colposcopy and acetic acid test: allow for the examination of the cervix and vagina. After the application of acetic acid solution; findings are graded according to degree of acetowhite lesion, surface contour, mosaic pattern, and punctuation;
- Biopsy: a critical part of colposcopy. If the biopsy results show pre-cancer (dysplasia) or cancer, then treatment is recommended. The dysplasia may be

mild, moderate or severe;

- DNA test (PCR, Southern Blot Hybridization, *In Situ* Hybridization): for molecular detection of HPV.

The prevalence of squamous intraepithelial lesions in HIV-seropositive patients is significantly higher than in the general female population, so seropositive patients should be screened frequently.

Treatments for HPV infection are limited, but some options include cryotherapy, loop electrosurgical excision procedures (LEEP), laser surgery, hysterectomy, chemotherapy and radiation therapy. Cervical pre-cancer can be successfully treated with cryotherapy or LEEP [23, 24].

2.2. Herpes Simplex Vírus (HSV)

Herpes simplex virus (HSV) exists as two types, 1 and 2 (HSV-1 and HSV-2) and causes a lasting infection with recurrent lesions. Generally, HSV-1 has been associated with orolabial diseases and HSV-2 is transmitted sexually and causes anogenital ulcers [25]. HSV-2 is a common co-infection among HIV-infected adults that is believed to accelerate HIV disease progression. HSV-2 active infection has high concentrations of active CD4+ T-cells (HIV target cells), facilitating mucosal layer rupture and HIV entry. Thus HSV-2 infection has a predisposition to increase viremia and transmissibility of HIV [26]. The virus becomes latent in the site of inoculation and HSV induces antibody and cell-mediated immune responses that modulate the severity of recurrent disease [27]. In immunocompromised individuals, such as those with HIV-1 infection, impaired immunity leads to more frequent and severe symptomatic and asymptomatic HSV reactivation [28].

Among HIV-1 infected individuals, the clinical presentation of symptomatic HSV-2 infection generally demonstrates vesicular and ulcerative lesions of the oral and anogenital areas and may be accompanied by systemic symptoms including fever, headache, myalgia, and viral meningitis. Often, genital reactivation may go unrecognized, because lesions are early or small. HIV-infected patients can also have frequent or persistent HSV lesions, often with extensive or deep ulcerations, particularly among those with low CD4 counts. In one study, the frequency of genital ulcer disease consistent with reactivation of genital herpes was found to increase in a stepwise fashion with declining CD4 counts [29, 30].

Notably, primary genital HSV-2 occurring in an HIV-1-infected person is an indicator of ongoing unsafe sexual practices and its course tends to be prolonged and more severe. More serious manifestations of HSV infection include esophagitis, meningoencephalitis, hepatitis, pneumonitis, retinal necrosis, and disseminated infection, all of which are relatively rare, even among those with advanced HIV-1 infection [30].

The clinical diagnosis of genital herpes should always include serotyping. The definitive diagnosis of genital herpes depends on the presence of HSV in the genital area, either by virus isolation or detection of antigen. Molecular diagnostic techniques are replacing viral culture and antigen detection can be used. The diagnosis of HSV infection will depend on the type of test, the quality of the specimen obtained, the ability of the laboratory to perform the test accurately, and the interpretation of the test results by the requesting clinician [31].

There is no cure for herpes, but antiviral medications can prevent or shorten outbreaks during the period the person takes the medication. Immunocompromised patients may have prolonged or severe episodes of HSV. Lesions caused by HSV are common among people with HIV infection and can be severe, painful and atypical. Suppressive or episodic therapy with oral antiviral agents is effective in reducing the clinical manifestations of HSV among HIV carriers (Table **1**) [32].

Table 1. Treatment schedule – co-infection HSV / HIV

Recommended regimens for Daily Suppressive Therapy for HIV carriers	Recommended regimens for Daily Episodic Infection for HIV carriers
Acyclovir 400–800 mg orally twice to three times a day	Acyclovir 400 mg orally three times a day for 5-10 days
Valacyclovir 500 mg orally twice a day	Valacyclovir 1 g orally twice a day for 5-10 days
Famciclovir 500 mg orally twice a day	Famciclovir 500 mg orally twice a day for 5-10 days

3. BACTERIAL GENITAL INFECTIONS

3.1. Syphilis

Syphilis is a sexually transmitted infection caused by the spirochete micro-organism *Treponema pallidum* [7]. Three stages of the disease are described: primary, secondary and tertiary syphilis. The first stage is asymptomatic in many cases but can also manifest as a small sore or ulcer. The secondary phase can include rashes anywhere on the body and small skin growths around the genital area. During the primary and secondary stages, it is easily transmissible through sexual contact. The tertiary phase follows a latent phase and can manifest with serious symptoms, causing damage to several organs, including heart, brain, bones and skin. The bacteria can be transmitted vertically and cause babies to be born with low birth weight, premature delivery and miscarriages [9]. The clinical stages of the disease are shown in Table **2**.

Table 2. Clinical Stage of Syphilis

Stage	Period	Symptoms
Primary	21 days after infection	Painless ulcer in genitals, skin and mouth
Secondary	4 – 8 weeks after primary infection	Body rash, headache, fever and lymphadenopathy
Tertiary	1 – 10 years after initial infection	Aortic insufficiency, aortic aneurysm, tabes dorsalis, loss of cortical function and altered mental state
Latent		
Early	One year after resolution of the primary or secondary lesions	Signs and symptoms usually disappear
Late	Unknown duration	Cardiovascular syphilis, neurosyphilis and syphilitic meningitis

The laboratory diagnosis of syphilis and the choice of the most appropriate laboratory tests should consider the evolutionary stage of the disease [9, 10]. A presumptive diagnosis of syphilis requires the use of two tests: a nontreponemal test (*i.e.,* Venereal Disease Research Laboratory [VDRL] or Rapid Plasma Reagin [RPR]) and a treponemal test (*i.e.,* fluorescent treponemal antibody absorbed [FTA-ABS] tests, the *T. pallidum* passive particle agglutination [TP-PA] assay, various enzyme immunoassays [EIAs], chemiluminescence immunoassays, immunoblots, or rapid treponemal assays).

Concomitant syphilis and HIV infections are particularly common among both women and men. On the other hand, HIV patients do not seem to present a higher risk of acquiring syphilis, even if it can progress much faster in HIV negative patients when acquired, and can be harder to treat, especially if there is a low CD4+ T-cells count [12, 33]. In this situation, the patient is at a high risk of developing neurosyphilis [34].

HIV and syphilis co-infection has a synergistic effect, characterized by both the elevation of HIV transmissibility and the atypical evolution of treponemic infection. The presence of sores in primary and secondary syphilis makes the HIV much easier to be transmitted [10].

Syphilis is one of the most common STIs, but its manifestations, especially its interaction with HIV, require further studies. Although there is effective treatment with the use of penicillin, the disease remains a major global health problem. Treatment guidelines are scarce, and there is a need for prospective studies that examine the course of the disease in HIV-infected patients [9].

Despite several advances in the understanding of the interaction between HIV infection and syphilis, the clinical treatment of co-infected patients remains challenging. Generally, the efficacy of therapy is monitored by the remission of symptoms and a decline in antibody titer. Co-infection with HIV can delay the decline in titer in both primary and secondary syphilis. The CDC guidelines suggest that the lack of a four-fold reduction in antibody titer at six months after primary and secondary syphilis therapy and within 12 to 24 months in latent syphilis with early high titers, identifies patients being at risk of treatment failure [1]. Recommended therapy for HIV-infected patients with syphilis at all stages is the same as for persons without HIV infection. Thus, persons with HIV and syphilis of unknown duration should receive three injections of benzathine penicillin, spaced at one-week intervals (Fig. **1**).

Recent syphilis: primary syphilis
Benzathine penicillin 2,400,000 IU, IM, single dose
Recent syphilis: recent secondary or latent syphilis (less than one year)
Benzathine penicillin 4,800,000 IU, IM, in two doses of 2,400,000 UI
Late syphilis: tertiary syphilis, latent late syphilis (with more than one year) and
latent syphilis of unknown time
Penicillin benzathine 7,200,000 IU, IM, in three doses of 2,400,000 UI
Individuals allergic to Penicillin
Doxycycline 100 mg, orally, 12/12 hours for 15 days or Ceftriaxone 1 g, intramuscularly or intravenously, once daily for 8 to 10 days.

Fig. (1). Syphilis Treatment Scheme.

3.2. *Chlamydia trachomatis*

Genital infection by *Chlamydia trachomatis* is one of the most prevalent bacterial sexually transmitted infections and most cases are found among young (15-24 years) women [35]. The infection by this agent is usually asymptomatic, preventing the diagnosis. The limited availability of specific laboratory tests in developing countries also complicates the diagnosis. If left untreated, the infection may evolve to pelvic inflammatory disease, chronic pelvic pain, tubal-factor infertility, ectopic pregnancy and cervical cancer. This infection can also lead to problems during pregnancy, including miscarriages, preterm labor and other effects on the child, such as conjunctivitis, nasopharyngitis and pneumonia [36, 37].

Previous studies have shown that *C. trachomatis* infection can increase the risk for HIV acquisition [37]. On the other hand, HIV may lead to a more aggressive chlamydia infection, and HIV positive women should be screened for *C. trachomatis* infection to prevent morbidity [38].

The diagnosis of chlamydial infection is usually done using serological methods, like ELISA. These methods are less sensitive than culture-based methods but have a rapid turnaround time and present lower requirements, making them more attractive as a point-of-care assay. Nucleic acid amplification tests present better sensitivity, specificity and can be multiplexed to detect other STIs. This method requires more complex facilities, it is also more expensive and requires specialized technicians, but its advantages should enable it to be more widely used in the near future.

C. trachomatis infection can be easily treated with antibiotics like tetracycline, doxycycline, or erythromycin (Table 3). Early detection and treatment of infected individuals are important to prevent adverse effects in those infected and also reduce transmission [39]. As young women are the most infected by this pathogen, it is important to screen this group for Chlamydia infection, even if they are asymptomatic.

Table 3. *Chlamydia trachomatis/HIV co-infection* treatment.

Recommended Regimen	
1 - Azithromycin	1 g orally in a single dose
2 – Doxycycline *	100 mg orally twice a day for 7 days
Alternative Regimen for women with HIV infection	
3 – Erythromycin base	500 mg orally four times a day for 7 days
4 - Erythromycin ethylsuccinate	800 mg orally four times a day for 7 days
5 – Levofloxacin *	500 mg orally daily for 7 days
6 –Ofloxacin *	300 mg orally twice a day for 7 days

* Not recommended during pregnancy

3.3. *Neisseria gonorrhoeae*

Neisseria gonorrhoeae is the etiological agent of gonorrhea, the second most frequently reported STI in the world. The bacteria typically colonizes the genital tract of men and women, but can also be found in rectal and oropharyngeal mucosa [35]. It is transmitted almost exclusively by sexual contact. The bacteria usually colonize the mucosal surface of lower urogenital tracts but can also be found in the rectum and pharynx. If left untreated, the disease can cause severe complications and morbidity. It can ascend to the upper genital tract and cause infections including pelvic inflammatory disease and related problems, including ectopic pregnancy and infertility. In newborns, it can cause ophthalmia neonatorum.

Women bearing gonorrhea have a significantly higher risk of HIV acquisition [40]. *N. gonorrhoeae* presence activates T CD4+ cells, rendering them more susceptible to HIV infection [41]. What is more, symptomatic gonorrhea is associated with an increased detection of viral particles in the plasma [42] and in genital secretion, potentially increasing the chance of transmission [43]. The low percentage of diagnostic screening in addition to inappropriate treatment maintain the bacterial STI chain-of-transmission, thus increasing STI and HIV transmission [44]. Both *N. gonorrhoeae* and *C. trachomatis* infections are important biologic markers of behavior that may expose others to HIV. Identification of HIV-infected women with CT or GC can help target preventive interventions such as promoting safer sexual practices [45, 46].

Gram-stained preparations can be examined to identify Gram-negative intracellular diplococcic in polymorphonuclear leukocytes, but the sensitivity is low in cervical samples and the specificity depends on the experience of the microscopist. Nucleic acid amplification tests are more sensitive, specific and can be multiplexed to detect other STIs. There are no immunological tests for antigen or antibody detection of gonorrhea with an acceptable performance.

Over the last decades, *N. gonorrhoeae* has developed resistance to sulfonamides, penicillin, tetracycline, ciprofloxacin, azithromycin and ceftriaxone. The emergence of this resistance and the absence of new treatments of gonorrhea have motivated the dual therapy protocols with ceftriaxone and azithromycin (Table **4**) [47]. Persons who are co-infected with HIV receive the same treatment regimen as those who are HIV negative.

Table 4. *Neisseria gonorrhoeae/HIV co-infection* treatment.

Recommended Regimen	
1 – Ceftriaxone PLUS	250 mg IM in a single dose
Azithromycin	1 g orally in a single dose

(Table 4) contd.....

Alternative Regimen	
2 – Cefixime PLUS	400 mg orally in a single dose
Azithromycin	1 g orally in a single dose

4. OTHER GENITAL INFECTIONS

4.1. Trichomonas vaginalis

Trichomonas vaginalis is the most common non-viral sexually transmitted pathogen. Its prevalence varies greatly depending on population and region, but is often greater than 10% in women, while the prevalence in men is much lower. This monoxenic protozoan is directly transmitted by sexual relations, and infects women more frequently, while men often act as a passive vector. The parasite binds to the vagina epithelial cells inducing a strong T CD4+ rich cellular immune response.

Although *T. vaginalis* acquisition has not been directly linked to HIV status, and it was recently shown that HIV infected women do not present higher rates of *T. vaginalis* infection, there still is an interaction between these pathogens. The presence of *T. vaginalis* in the vagina increases the rate of HIV that is acquired, probably because of the increase in T CD4+ leukocytes and the constant epithelial cell shedding and micro fissures it causes [48]. There is also the possibility that the protozoan increases the virus shedding, potentially increasing the chance of transmission, although there is still no definitive answer to this question.

The classical diagnosis method is using wet saline mounts, where motile parasites can be observed. This method relies on the expertise of the reader and presents low sensitivity. Cultures using specific medium are more sensitive but are more laborious and time consuming. Nowadays there are many rapid point-of-care tests that can quickly diagnose *T. vaginalis* infections in both women and men [49]. DNA amplification methods are the most sensitive tests, they are moderately priced but require specialized technicians.

There are indications that the single dose metronidazole treatment of *T. vaginalis* present a higher failure rate in HIV+ women [50]. Reinfection seems to be particularly high in this group, suggesting that the treatment does not present the same efficiency found in HIV- women, and indicating that a multi dose treatment might be more efficient [51, 52]. In any case, rescreening is important to exclude treatment failure. Other drugs include tinidazole and secnidazole, both related to metronidazole. Although tinidazole presents a higher clearance rate and fewer side effects, it is considerably more expensive, and thus metronidazole remains the first drug of choice (Table **5**).

Table 5. *Trichomonas vaginalis /HIV co-infection* **treatment.**

Recommended Regimen	
1 - Metronidazole	2 g orally in a single dose
2 - Tinidazole	2 g orally in a single dose
Alternative Regimen for women with HIV infection	
3 - Metronidazole	500 mg twice a day for 7 days

CONCLUSION

The introduction of ART has improved the quality of life of people living with HIV. It has also improved their sexual lives with the downside of rendering condom use not so imperative in the prevention of HIV transmission. It is important to note that even if the HIV viral levels are under control, the transmission of other STIs are still possible and could be prevented by condom use. Increasing rates of sex without condoms in this group has also increased the transmission of other sexually transmitted diseases. The transmission is facilitated because of the synergistic effect between HIV and other STIs, as discussed above, reinforcing the idea that condom use should not be abandoned. It is well established that many STIs are more easily transmissible when HIV is also present. The return of many of these STIs can be partially attributed to this synergistic effect. It is also important to consider the fact that many individuals infected with STIs are asymptomatic with what has been called a "hidden infection" [53].

For these reasons, the screening for other STIs in HIV positive patients should be improved and done regularly. CDC recommends the minimum of annual STI testing of HIV+ patients [54], but recent studies indicate that screening is far from ideal, even in the United States [55]. HIV infected individuals present higher rates of STI, which also suggests the persistence of high risk sexual behavior [56]. Prevention counseling in primary care settings can decrease subsequent STIs in HIV+ individuals and influence patients to change to achievable risk-reducing behavior [54]. Screening is particularly imperative in those cases where the synergistic effects of HIV and other STI agents lead to a more potent version of the disease that can lead to greater morbidity. In these cases, quick treatment in the early stages can prevent this morbidity, greatly enhancing the quality of life of the patient.

CONSENT FOR PUBLICATION

Not applicable.

CONFLICT OF INTEREST

The authors declare no conflict of interest, financial or otherwise.

ACKNOWLEDGEMENT

Declared none.

REFERENCES

[1]   Al-Jabri AA. Mechanisms of host resistance against HIV infection and progression to AIDS. Sultan Qaboos Univ Med J 2007; 7(2): 82-96.
[PMID: 21748089]

[2]   Hariri S, McKenna MT. Epidemiology of human immunodeficiency virus in the United States. Clin Microbiol Rev 2007; 20(3): 478-88.
[http://dx.doi.org/10.1128/CMR.00006-07] [PMID: 17630336]

[3]   Cohen MS, Chen YQ, McCauley M, *et al.* HPTN 052 Study Team. Antiretroviral Therapy for the Prevention of HIV-1 Transmission. N Engl J Med 2016; 375(9): 830-9.
[http://dx.doi.org/10.1056/NEJMoa1600693] [PMID: 27424812]

[4]   Fidler S, Anderson J, Azad Y, *et al.* Position statement on the use of antiretroviral therapy to reduce HIV transmission, January 2013: the British HIV Association (BHIVA) and the Expert Advisory Group on AIDS (EAGA). HIV Med 2013; 14(5): 259-62.
[http://dx.doi.org/10.1111/hiv.12025] [PMID: 23489936]

[5]   Albert J, Berglund T, Gisslén M, *et al.* Risk of HIV transmission from patients on antiretroviral therapy: a position statement from the Public Health Agency of Sweden and the Swedish Reference Group for Antiviral Therapy. Scand J Infect Dis 2014; 46(10): 673-7.
[http://dx.doi.org/10.3109/00365548.2014.926565] [PMID: 25073537]

[6]   Marrazzo JM, Dombrowski JC, Mayer KH. Sexually transmitted infections in the era of antiretroviral-based HIV prevention: Priorities for discovery research, implementation science, and community involvement. PLoS Med 2018; 15(1): e1002485.
[http://dx.doi.org/10.1371/journal.pmed.1002485] [PMID: 29320494]

[7]   Abdool Karim Q, Sibeko S, Baxter C. Preventing HIV infection in women: a global health imperative. Clin Infect Dis 2010; 50 (Suppl. 3): S122-9.
[http://dx.doi.org/10.1086/651483] [PMID: 20397940]

[8]   Berretta M, Caraglia M, Martellotta F, *et al.* Drug-drug interactions based on pharmacogenetic profile between highly active antiretroviral therapy and antiblastic chemotherapy in cancer patients with HIV infection. Front Pharmacol 2016; 7: 71.
[http://dx.doi.org/10.3389/fphar.2016.00071] [PMID: 27065862]

[9]   Singh AE, Romanowski B. Syphilis: review with emphasis on clinical, epidemiologic, and some biologic features. Clin Microbiol Rev 1999; 12(2): 187-209.
[PMID: 10194456]

[10]   Nwankwo A, Okuonghae D. Mathematical Analysis of the Transmission Dynamics of HIV Syphilis Co-infection in the Presence of Treatment for Syphilis. Bull Math Biol 2018; 80(3): 437-92.
[http://dx.doi.org/10.1007/s11538-017-0384-0] [PMID: 29282597]

[11]   Cubie HA. Diseases associated with human papillomavirus infection. Virology 2013; 445(1-2): 21-34.
[http://dx.doi.org/10.1016/j.virol.2013.06.007] [PMID: 23932731]

[12]   Doorbar J, Egawa N, Griffin H, Kranjec C, Murakami I. Human papillomavirus molecular biology and disease association. Rev Med Virol 2015; 25 (Suppl. 1): 2-23.
[http://dx.doi.org/10.1002/rmv.1822] [PMID: 25752814]

[13]   Doorbar J. The papillomavirus life cycle. J Clin Virol 2005; 32 (Suppl. 1): S7-S15.
        [http://dx.doi.org/10.1016/j.jcv.2004.12.006] [PMID: 15753007]

[14]   Hsueh P-R. Human papillomavirus, genital warts, and vaccines. J Microbiol Immunol Infect 2009;
        42(2): 101-6.

[15]   Burd EM. Human papillomavirus and cervical cancer. Clin Microbiol Rev 2003; 16(1): 1-17.
        [http://dx.doi.org/10.1128/CMR.16.1.1-17.2003] [PMID: 12525422]

[16]   Palefsky JM, Holly EA, Ralston ML, Jay N. Prevalence and risk factors for human papillomavirus
        infection of the anal canal in human immunodeficiency virus (HIV)-positive and HIV-negative
        homosexual men. J Infect Dis 1998; 177(2): 361-7.
        [http://dx.doi.org/10.1086/514194] [PMID: 9466522]

[17]   Palefsky JM, Holly EA, Ralston ML, Greenblatt RM, Greenblatt RM. Da Costa M. Prevalence and
        risk factors for anal human papillomavirus infection in human immunodeficiency virus (HIV)-positive
        and high-risk HIV-negative women. J Infect Dis 2001; 183(3): 383-91.
        [http://dx.doi.org/10.1086/318071] [PMID: 11133369]

[18]   Lissouba P, Van de Perre P, Auvert B. Association of genital human papillomavirus infection with
        HIV acquisition: a systematic review and meta-analysis. Sex Transm Infect 2013; 89(5): 350-6.
        [http://dx.doi.org/10.1136/sextrans-2011-050346] [PMID: 23761216]

[19]   Ghebre RG, Grover S, Xu MJ, Chuang LT, Simonds H. Cervical cancer control in HIV-infected
        women: Past, present and future. Gynecol Oncol Rep 2017; 21: 101-8.
        [http://dx.doi.org/10.1016/j.gore.2017.07.009] [PMID: 28819634]

[20]   Franceschi S, Lise M, Clifford GM, *et al.* Swiss HIV Cohort Study. Changing patterns of cancer
        incidence in the early- and late-HAART periods: the Swiss HIV Cohort Study. Br J Cancer 2010;
        103(3): 416-22.
        [http://dx.doi.org/10.1038/sj.bjc.6605756] [PMID: 20588274]

[21]   De Vuyst H, Mugo NR, Chung MH, *et al.* Prevalence and determinants of human papillomavirus
        infection and cervical lesions in HIV-positive women in Kenya. Br J Cancer 2012; 107(9): 1624-30.
        [http://dx.doi.org/10.1038/bjc.2012.441] [PMID: 23033006]

[22]   Corbeau P, Reynes J. Immune reconstitution under antiretroviral therapy: the new challenge in HIV-1
        infection. Blood 2011; 117(21): 5582-90.
        [http://dx.doi.org/10.1182/blood-2010-12-322453] [PMID: 21403129]

[23]   Moore DH. Chemotherapy for recurrent cervical carcinoma. Curr Opin Oncol 2006; 18(5): 516-9.
        [http://dx.doi.org/10.1097/01.cco.0000239893.21161.51] [PMID: 16894302]

[24]   Chuang LT, Temin S, Camacho R, *et al.* Management and Care of Women With Invasive Cervical
        Cancer: American Society of Clinical Oncology Resource-Stratified Clinical Practice Guideline. J
        Glob Oncol 2016; 2(5): 311-40.
        [http://dx.doi.org/10.1200/JGO.2016.003954] [PMID: 28717717]

[25]   Pereira VSS, Moizeis RNC, Fernandes TAAM, Araújo JMG, Meissner RV, Fernandes JV. Herpes
        simplex virus type 1 is the main cause of genital herpes in women of Natal, Brazil. Eur J Obstet
        Gynecol Reprod Biol 2012; 161(2): 190-3.
        [http://dx.doi.org/10.1016/j.ejogrb.2011.12.006] [PMID: 22424592]

[26]   Looker KJ, Elmes JAR, Gottlieb SL, *et al.* Effect of HSV-2 infection on subsequent HIV acquisition:
        an updated systematic review and meta-analysis. Lancet Infect Dis 2017; 17(12): 1303-16.
        [http://dx.doi.org/10.1016/S1473-3099(17)30405-X] [PMID: 28843576]

[27]   Tan DH-S, Murphy K, Shah P, Walmsley SL. Herpes simplex virus type 2 and HIV disease
        progression: a systematic review of observational studies. BMC Infect Dis 2013; 13: 502.
        [http://dx.doi.org/10.1186/1471-2334-13-502] [PMID: 24164861]

[28]   Strick LB, Wald A, Celum C. Management of herpes simplex virus type 2 infection in HIV type 1-

infected persons. Clin Infect Dis 2006; 43(3): 347-56.
[http://dx.doi.org/10.1086/505496] [PMID: 16804851]

[29]   McClelland RS, Lavreys L, Katingima C, *et al.* Contribution of HIV-1 infection to acquisition of sexually transmitted disease: a 10-year prospective study. J Infect Dis 2005; 191(3): 333-8.
[http://dx.doi.org/10.1086/427262] [PMID: 15633091]

[30]   Tan DHS, Raboud JM, Kaul R, *et al.* Herpes simplex virus type 2 coinfection does not accelerate CD4 count decline in untreated HIV infection. Clin Infect Dis 2013; 57(3): 448-57.
[http://dx.doi.org/10.1093/cid/cit208] [PMID: 23572481]

[31]   Singh A, Preiksaitis J, Ferenczy A, Romanowski B. The laboratory diagnosis of herpes simplex virus infections. Can J Infect Dis Med Microbiol 2005; 16(2): 92-8.
[http://dx.doi.org/10.1155/2005/318294] [PMID: 18159535]

[32]   Posavad CM, Wald A, Kuntz S, *et al.* Frequent reactivation of herpes simplex virus among HIV--infected patients treated with highly active antiretroviral therapy. J Infect Dis 2004; 190(4): 693-6.
[http://dx.doi.org/10.1086/422755] [PMID: 15272395]

[33]   Chiasson MANN, Ellerbrock TV, Bush TJ, Sun XW, Wright TC Jr. Increased prevalence of vulvovaginal condyloma and vulvar intraepithelial neoplasia in women infected with the human immunodeficiency virus. Obstet Gynecol 1997; 89(5 Pt 1): 690-4.
[http://dx.doi.org/10.1016/S0029-7844(97)00069-0] [PMID: 9166302]

[34]   Sadeghani K, Kallini JR, Khachemoune A. Neurosyphilis in a Man with Human Immunodeficiency Virus. J Clin Aesthet Dermatol 2014; 7(8): 35-40.

[35]   Chan PA, Robinette A, Montgomery M, *et al.* Extragenital Infections Caused by Chlamydia trachomatis and Neisseria gonorrhoeae: A Review of the Literature. Infect Dis Obstet Gynecol 2016; 2016: 5758387.
[http://dx.doi.org/10.1155/2016/5758387] [PMID: 27366021]

[36]   Land JA, Van Bergen JEAM, Morré SA, Postma MJ. Epidemiology of Chlamydia trachomatis infection in women and the cost-effectiveness of screening. Hum Reprod Update 2010; 16(2): 189-204.
[http://dx.doi.org/10.1093/humupd/dmp035] [PMID: 19828674]

[37]   Bhattar S, Bhalla P, Chadha S, Tripathi R, Kaur R, Sardana K. Chlamydia trachomatis infection in HIV-infected women: need for screening by a sensitive and specific test. Infect Dis Obstet Gynecol 2013; 2013: 960769.
[http://dx.doi.org/10.1155/2013/960769] [PMID: 24382941]

[38]   Thomas K, Simms I. Chlamydia trachomatis in subfertile women undergoing uterine instrumentation. How we can help in the avoidance of iatrogenic pelvic inflammatory disease? Hum Reprod 2002; 17(6): 1431-2.
[http://dx.doi.org/10.1093/humrep/17.6.1431] [PMID: 12042255]

[39]   Haggerty CL, Gottlieb SL, Taylor BD, Low N, Xu F, Ness RB. Risk of sequelae after *Chlamydia trachomatis* genital infection in women. J Infect Dis 2010; 201 (Suppl. 2): S134-55.
[http://dx.doi.org/10.1086/652395] [PMID: 20470050]

[40]   Mlisana K, Naicker N, Werner L, *et al.* Symptomatic vaginal discharge is a poor predictor of sexually transmitted infections and genital tract inflammation in high-risk women in South Africa. J Infect Dis 2012; 206(1): 6-14.
[http://dx.doi.org/10.1093/infdis/jis298] [PMID: 22517910]

[41]   Ding J, Rapista A, Teleshova N, *et al.* Neisseria gonorrhoeae enhances HIV-1 infection of primary resting CD4+ T cells through TLR2 activation. J Immunol 2010; 184(6): 2814-24.
[http://dx.doi.org/10.4049/jimmunol.0902125] [PMID: 20147631]

[42]   Anzala AO, Simonsen JN, Kimani J, *et al.* Acute sexually transmitted infections increase human immunodeficiency virus type 1 plasma viremia, increase plasma type 2 cytokines, and decrease CD4

cell counts. J Infect Dis 2000; 182(2): 459-66.
[http://dx.doi.org/10.1086/315733] [PMID: 10915076]

[43]   Cohen MS, Hoffman IF, Royce RA, *et al.* AIDSCAP Malawi Research Group. Reduction of concentration of HIV-1 in semen after treatment of urethritis: implications for prevention of sexual transmission of HIV-1. Lancet 1997; 349(9069): 1868-73.
[http://dx.doi.org/10.1016/S0140-6736(97)02190-9] [PMID: 9217758]

[44]   Travassos AG, Xavier-Souza E, Netto E, *et al.* Anogenital infection by Chlamydia trachomatis and Neisseria gonorrhoeae in HIV-infected men and women in Salvador, Brazil. Braz J Infect Dis 2016; 20(6): 569-75.
[http://dx.doi.org/10.1016/j.bjid.2016.09.004] [PMID: 27765581]

[45]   Mestecky J, Moldoveanu Z, Smith PD, Hel Z, Alexander RC. Mucosal immunology of the genital and gastrointestinal tracts and HIV-1 infection. J Reprod Immunol 2009; 83(1-2): 196-200.
[http://dx.doi.org/10.1016/j.jri.2009.07.005] [PMID: 19853927]

[46]   Stahlman S, Hirz AE, Stirland A, Guerry S, Gorbach PM, Javanbakht M. Contextual factors surrounding anal intercourse in women: Implications for sexually transmitted infection/HIV prevention. Sex Transm Dis 2015; 42(7): 364-8.
[http://dx.doi.org/10.1097/OLQ.0000000000000303] [PMID: 26222748]

[47]   Costa-Lourenço APRD, Barros Dos Santos KT, Moreira BM, Fracalanzza SEL, Bonelli RR. Antimicrobial resistance in Neisseria gonorrhoeae: history, molecular mechanisms and epidemiological aspects of an emerging global threat. Braz J Microbiol 2017; 48(4): 617-28.
[http://dx.doi.org/10.1016/j.bjm.2017.06.001] [PMID: 28754299]

[48]   Thurman AR, Doncel GF. Innate immunity and inflammatory response to Trichomonas vaginalis and bacterial vaginosis: relationship to HIV acquisition. Am J Reprod Immunol 2011; 65(2): 89-98.
[http://dx.doi.org/10.1111/j.1600-0897.2010.00902.x] [PMID: 20678168]

[49]   Gaydos CA, Klausner JD, Pai NP, Kelly H, Coltart C, Peeling RW. Rapid and point-of-care tests for the diagnosis of *Trichomonas vaginalis* in women and men, Sex. Sex Transm Infect 2017; 93(S4): S31-5.

[50]   Kissinger P, Secor WE, Leichliter JS, *et al.* Early repeated infections with Trichomonas vaginalis among HIV-positive and HIV-negative women. Clin Infect Dis 2008; 46(7): 994-9.
[http://dx.doi.org/10.1086/529149] [PMID: 18444815]

[51]   Gatski M, Martin DH, Levison J, *et al.* The influence of bacterial vaginosis on the response to Trichomonas vaginalis treatment among HIV-infected women. Sex Transm Infect 2011; 87(3): 205-8.
[http://dx.doi.org/10.1136/sti.2010.046441] [PMID: 21278401]

[52]   Adamski A, Clark RA, Mena L, *et al.* The influence of ART on the treatment of Trichomonas vaginalis among HIV-infected women. Clin Infect Dis 2014; 59(6): 883-7.
[http://dx.doi.org/10.1093/cid/ciu401] [PMID: 24917661]

[53]   Tracking the Hidden Epidemics. Trends in STDs in the United States 2000. www.cdc.gov/std/trends2000/trends2000.pdf

[54]   Burstein GR, Workowski KA. Sexually Transmitted Diseases Treatment Guidelines, 2015. MMWR Recomm Rep 2015; 64(RR-03): 1-137.
[http://dx.doi.org/10.1097/00008480-200308000-00006]

[55]   Landovitz RJ, Gildner JL, Leibowitz AA. Sexually Transmitted Infection Testing of HIV-Positive Medicare and Medicaid Enrollees Falls Short of Guidelines. Sex Transm Dis 2018; 45(1): 8-13.
[http://dx.doi.org/10.1097/OLQ.0000000000000695] [PMID: 29240633]

[56]   Castro JG, Alcaide ML. High Rates of STIs in HIV-Infected Patients Attending an STI Clinic. South Med J 2016; 109(1): 1-4.
[http://dx.doi.org/10.14423/SMJ.0000000000000389] [PMID: 26741862]

SUBJECT INDEX

A

Abacavir 4, 6, 7
AC field 48
Acid 71, 72, 74, 82, 88, 97, 112
  2,4-difluorobenzoic 71, 72
  Aspartic 112
Acquired immunodeficiency syndrome
  (AIDS) 2, 5, 30, 36, 61, 63, 105, 114,
  120, 129, 138, 140
  virus 138
Active 41, 42, 63, 84, 99
  pharmaceutical intermediates (APIs) 63, 84,
  99
  targeting ability 41, 42
Acyclovir 142
Adverse events, drug-related 125
Agents, bioactive 50
AIDS-related complex (ARC) 120
Alternating current (AC) 48, 49
Amide 19, 87, 88, 89, 120
  vinylogous 87
Amidoxine 66, 67
Aminonitrile 65, 67
Amphoterism 44, 45
Amprenavir 1, 2, 4, 12, 13, 23, 27
Antibiotics, quinolone 71
Antibodies 43, 122, 141
Antiretroviral drugs 4, 35, 62, 82, 115, 129
  approved 82, 115
API synthesis 63, 85, 95
Apoptosis 37
ARV drugs 39, 42, 43, 52
Aryl 16, 17, 74, 92, 93
  alkyl groups 16, 17
  isocyanate, generated 92, 93
  lithium species 74
Astrocytes 35, 36, 37, 39, 47, 112
Atazanavir 63, 96, 98, 99
ATP-binding cassette (ABC) 39
Azithromycin 145, 146, 147

B

Binding interactions 7, 12, 14, 17, 19, 26, 29,
  30
Blood-brain barrier (BBB) 34, 35, 36, 37, 38,
  39, 40, 42, 43, 45, 46, 47
Brain-derived neurotropic factor (BDNF) 47
Bromide, 3-chloro-2-fluorobenzyl zinc 72, 73

C

Carbamates 2, 19, 23, 24, 25
  tetrahydrofuran 23, 24
Carbonate, cesium 23, 24
CC chemokines 113, 114
CCR5 4, 5, 114, 115
  co-receptor 4, 5
  function of 114, 115
CCR5 113, 114, 115, 120, 121, 123, 127, 128
  antagonists 113, 114, 115, 123
  cell lines 128
  co-receptor 120, 121
  inhibitors 115
  surface expression 127
CD4+ T-lymphocytes 2, 3
Ceftriaxone 144, 146
Cell adhesion 108, 109, 127
Cells, inflammatory-response 43
Cellular carrier 43
Cenicriviroc 118
  -treated participants 118
  VFs 118
Chlamydia trachomatis 138, 144
Core, hydroxypyrimidinone 66
Coreceptors signaling 109
Corona effect 51
Cross-reactivity 11
Cryotherapy 141
CXCR4 Antagonists 123, 124
Cyclic sulfonamides 1, 2, 14, 16, 17, 18, 23,
  24, 29

www.ingramcontent.com/pod-product-compliance
Lightning Source LLC
Chambersburg PA
CBHW041708210326
41598CB00007B/581